Management and Security of Health Information on Mobile Devices

Claudia Tessier, MEd, RHIA

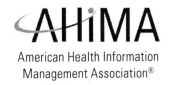

AHiMA
American Health Information
Management Association®

ISBN: 978-1-58426-230-5

AHIMA Product No.: AB108009

AHIMA Staff:

Claire Blondeau, MBA, Senior Editor

Cynthia Douglas, Developmental Editor

Katie Greenock, Editorial and Production Coordinator

Ashley Sullivan, Assistant Editor

Ken Zielske, Director of Publications

All information contained within this book, including Web sites and regulatory information, was current and valid as of the date of publication. However, Web page addresses and the information on them may change or disappear at any time and for any number of reasons. The user is encouraged to perform his or her own general Web searches to locate any site addresses listed here that are no longer valid.

This book is not intended to be a substitute for legal advice, and its recommendations should not be adopted without review by an organization's legal counsel to ensure compliance with federal, state, and local laws as well as institutional policies and procedures.

American Health Information Management Association

233 North Michigan Avenue, 21st floor

Chicago, Illinois 60601-5800

ahima.org

CONTENTS

ABOUT THE AUTHOR

Claudia Tessier, MEd, RHIA, is president of mHealth Initiative, a not-for-profit organization that promotes the adoption of mobile devices and applications in healthcare as the future conduits of interoperability for essential health information and as a means of enabling participatory health. From 2006 to 2009, Tessier was vice president of Medical Records Institute, where she was responsible for program development and delivery as well as executive management of the institute's mission to promote and enhance the movement toward electronic medical records (EMR), e-health, mobile health, and related information technologies. Tessier earned her registered records administrator (RRA) credential through the U.S. Public Health Service (USPHS) program in Baltimore, MD in 1979 and served as assistant medical records administrator at the USPHS Hospital in Nassau Bay, TX, from 1979 to 1980. She was an assistant professor of medical records administration at the University of Illinois Medical Center, Chicago from 1980 to 1982, and then at the University of Wisconsin–Milwaukee in fall 1982. In 1983 she was appointed director of education of the American Association for Medical Transcription (AAMT), advancing to the CEO position in 1984 and served in that position until 2001. From 2001 to 2006 she was executive director of the Mobile Healthcare Alliance (MoHCA). In 2002, Tessier was appointed as co-chair of the Continuity of Care Record (CCR) Task Group, which is sponsored by ASTM International's E31 Committee on Healthcare Informatics, the Massachusetts Medical Society, the American Academy of Family Practice, the American Academy of Pediatrics, the American Medical Association, and other organizations. In 2002 and 2003, Tessier served as vice chair of the American National Standards Institute's Healthcare Informatics Standards Board (ANSI-HISB), the predecessor of the current Health Information Technology Standards Board (ANSI-HITSP). Tessier authored the first edition (1995) of *The AAMT Book of Style for Medical Transcription*, and she is preparing the fourth edition of *The Surgical Word Book*, first published in 1981. She is an internationally recognized expert, speaker, writer, and consultant on healthcare documentation, the CCR, electronic medical records, and mHealth.

Acknowledgements

The author thanks C. Peter Waegemann of mHealth Initiative for his valuable expertise, contributions to, and review of this book and for his dedication to the goals of mHealth. She also thanks Fred Tessier for his valuable assistance in the book's preparation.

INTRODUCTION

Nearly 90 percent of the U.S. population has at least one cell phone, and almost one in five people have replaced their landlines with a cell phone. And these numbers are growing. When people leave their homes, taking their cell phones is as important as taking their wallets. The rise of the computer began changing our society in the last quarter of the 20th century. In the 21st century, it is the mobile phone that is dramatically impacting how we communicate, find our way, and select an eating place, just to mention a few of the thousands of applications available for cell phones. The evolution of the cell phone into an extension of the Internet has given this technology an unprecedented surge. The cell phone "tsunami" happened faster than the development of any previous technology, and it is impossible to predict where the cell phone as a personal and professional communication device will lead.

What does this mean for healthcare and the health information management (HIM) profession? While most hospitals banned mobile phones with "no-cell phone" policies only a few years ago, such policies have mostly been discarded or modified. Cell phones are transitioning from forbidden gadgets to prized tools for healthcare professionals and patients. This means that HIM professionals must prepare themselves to develop and administer policies and procedures to address the security of protected health information (PHI) that is accessed, stored, or communicated through mobile devices (mDevices). This will also mean strengthening their ties to information technology (IT) and security professionals, as well as to clinicians, legal counsel, C-level executives, department heads, patients themselves, and others.

This book provides an overview of the many mobile applications that will directly impact HIM professionals as well as applications particularly applicable to and of interest to patients, clinicians, administrative personnel, emergency technicians, nurses, public health professionals, and numerous others. This new territory of mobile functionalities is mapped into 12 application clusters, within which numerous applications will lead to major restructuring of the information and communication flow.

In this book, the reader can expect to find information on a wide range of applications already in use in 2010 and an outlook of what is to come, to the extent that this dynamic industry can be predicted and anticipated. At a time when costs and efficiencies are focal points in most healthcare organizations and throughout our society, mobile health (mHealth) offers a solution through healthcare that is based on new communication patterns. Indeed, all these changes may be summed up as the mHealth revolution.

This book points out that the traditional cell phone could not have had such an impact. However, today's cell phones include numerous other functionalities. Therefore, the term cell phone itself is outdated. Rather, they are mobile phones, mobile computers, cameras, identification devices, personal assistants, banking devices, and much more; that is, they are smartphones. In short, we are entering the historic era of mobile devices in healthcare, and these devices are now better called mDevices, because voice communi-cation is only a small part of their functionality and potential impact on healthcare.

While the emphasis in this text is on cell phones, it is important to remember that mDevices also include larger, portable wireless devices such as laptops, notebooks, netbooks, and tablets, as well as smaller, removable devices, such as CDs and USB drives. Further, just as cell phones have added data communication to their functionalities, the larger mDevices have added voice communication through Voice over Internet Protocol (VoIP). Since VoIP is also available on desktop computers and cell phones, these larger mDevices in a sense straddle the two markets. Nevertheless, it is the cell phone, or more accurately the smartphone, that is the leader in electronic communications (eCommunication) by offering both the greatest portability (in a pocket, purse, or hand) and the farthest-ranging functionality through the tens of thousands of applications that they offer and that users are enthusiastically adopting. That said, keep in mind that, despite our focus on the smartphone, we will regularly use the term mDevice, and further, that the concerns and controls that we emphasize for smartphones apply to other mDevices as well, according to their ability to receive, store, allow access to, and communicate PHI. These concerns and controls include electromagnetic interference, authentication, data integrity, confidentially, security, interoperability, brownouts, and clinical grade goals, as well as risk management and managing multiple devices over multiple networks.

It must be emphasized that all that mDevices offer healthcare could not have its greatest impact without the rise of a new paradigm—participatory health. The active participation of people, patients, healthcare professionals, payers, public health professionals, and many others is poised to create a historic change in healthcare, with the mDevice as its enabler and the catalyst for the mHealth revolution. Participatory health could not be achieved without the rise of mDevices and the development of new communication systems. And mDevices would not have such an impact without the rise of this new healthcare structure that depends on the active participation of all healthcare participants, with the patient at the center.

This overview of this exploding field is intended to identify new opportunities for professional development and roles for HIM professionals and to encourage them to be proactive in meeting the challenges they bring. It also aims to help HIM professionals and others to adapt the traditional procedures and approaches of health information management developed for legal and professional documentation in the age of paper and electronic medical records (EMRs) to this new field of mobile wireless communication. New guidelines and policies need to be developed in response to many mobile applications. Such policies are described in general terms because the field is so new that no consensus yet exists on details. National standards remain to be developed.

Finally, this book makes the point that mHealth will be much more demanding and exciting to HIM professionals than EMRs and paper records. Systems must be reorganized and new workflows implemented. These changes and opportunities will give HIM a new meaning and a new place in healthcare, as health information management systems increasingly become health communication management systems. Certainly, they will reinforce and expand the opportunities and necessity for HIM professionals to work in tandem with health information technology and bioengineering specialists and others to assure that their unique qualifications, interests, and responsibilities converge to maximize the synergy their cooperation can bring to the adoption and management of mHealth.

Note: Throughout this book, the author has used the terms electronic medical record (EMR) and electronic health record (EHR) according to the definitions prepared by the National Alliance for Health Information Technology (NAHIT) for the Department of Health and Human Services, Office of the National Coordinator for Health Information Technology: An EMR is "an electronic record of health-related information on an individual that can be created gathered, managed, and consulted by authorized clinicians and staff within one health care organization", in contrast to an EHR, which is "an electronic record of health-related information that conforms to nationally recognized interoperability standards and can be created, managed, and consulted by authorized clinicians and staff across more than one health care organization." (NAHIT 2008)

Note: This book is not intended to be a substitute for legal advice, and its recommendations should not be adopted without review by an organization's legal counsel to ensure compliance with federal, state, and local laws as well as institutional policies and procedures.

CHAPTER 1

Mobile Wireless Devices and Mobile Health (mHealth)

Introduction

Cell phones have come a long way since the turn of the century. Today's mobile devices (mDevices) range from smartphones to highly functional tablets and wireless band aids that transmit vital signs to an mDevice or electronic medical record (EMR)*. Companies have created a number of names for such devices, some proprietary, and some generic (for example, communicator, companion, touch phone, iPhone, Blackberry, and Android). In healthcare they are generally referred to as mobile devices or mDevices, and they are increasingly becoming a routine part of any health information system. Over time, they will likely become essential companions for anyone involved in healthcare, from patients and providers to pharmacies and payers, and more.

Indeed, all signs indicate that handheld mDevices and wireless communication are creating a revolution in healthcare and health informatics, and it is important that health information management (HIM) professionals incorporate this evolving phenomenon into their work. HIM and other health information specialists must recognize and understand the potential that such new devices and systems hold to improve the quality and efficiency of healthcare, and at the same time they must become familiar with the potential threats of such systems and devices to the established principles of health information management.

---

*Throughout this book, the author has used the terms electronic medical record (EMR) and electronic health record (EHR) according to the definitions prepared by the National Alliance for Health Information Technology (NAHIT) for the Department of Health and Human Services, Office of the National Coordinator for Health Information Technology: An EMR is "an electronic record of health-related information on an individual that can be created gathered, managed, and consulted by authorized clinicians and staff within one health care organization", in contrast to an EHR, which is "an electronic record of health-related information that conforms to nationally recognized interoperability standards and can be created, managed, and consulted by authorized clinicians and staff across more than one health care organization." (NAHIT 2008)

For decades, HIM professionals have guided clinicians and others involved in the care process in creating legal and permanent documentation. As we enter the new era of mobile and wireless communication, the principles that governed paper records must be applied to these new systems. The technologies for documenting on an mDevice continue to evolve. For example, mDevices are anticipated that will enable a physician to project an enlarged, functional image of his keyboard onto a flat surface such his office desk or a tray next to a patient's bed, allowing easier data entry. Whatever the form of documentation, authentication, security, auditing, data integrity, and confidentiality are just a few of the issues that must be addressed when a provider organization incorporates the use of mobile phones into its communication system. Thus, it is important to understand the conditions that enable clinicians and others to use these devices and systems to the fullest benefit for patients, caregivers, provider institutions, payers, and others, addressing them as powerful enablers and managing their potential threats.

What Are Mobile Wireless Devices?

When telephones were invented almost a century and a half ago, their ability to allow two people to speak to one another through a wire challenged belief. Today, speaking to another person over a wire is taken for granted, and telephony developments are moving at an ever-increasing pace and providing previously unimagined connectivity. "Speaking through the air," or speaking without wiring, is the communication miracle of our times.

The ability to transmit voice wirelessly was first demonstrated in the 1970s. The enabling device was huge and weighed several pounds. Since then, mobile phones have shrunk in size and weight, while offering increasingly powerful features, which are being widely adopted. At the end of 2008, more than four billion mobile phones were in use worldwide (3G Americas 2008). Over 270 million of these are in the United States, representing a wireless penetration of 87 percent of the U.S. population (CTIA 2008). A Centers for Disease Control (CDC) report shows "wireless only households made up 14.7 percent of U.S. households in 2007" (Blumberg et al. 2009). A related press release emphasizes the importance of these findings because it means that adults with only cell phones are being omitted from most of their large surveys, which are done on calls to landline phones. The press release noted, "A recent report found that 17.5 percent of U.S. homes had only wireless telephones during the first half of 2008...." (CDC Online Newsroom 2009).

Mobile wireless devices include cell phones with built-in computers, Internet browsers, cameras, and other capabilities. What started out as a voice-enabled cell phone evolved into a personal digital assistant that also functions as an appointment calendar, contact database, and more. Add to this the capability to transmit not only voice but also data, and you have something like a mobile, virtual fax machine. But the real breakthrough came with the addition of user-friendly browsers that enable easy Internet surfing, which allows quick and easy searching for any information. This brought the term smartphone into play, and now smartphones have greater functionalities, such as global positioning systems (GPS) that allow you to find your way while driving or walking. In naming these devices, manufacturers have tried to keep up with their evolving functionalities, whether by using proprietary terminology (for example, iPhone or Android) or generic terminology (for example, personal digital assistant [PDA] or smartphone). Currently, the most common and appropriate term for the universe of these devices is mobile device, or more commonly, mDevice.

Wireless phones represent the most rapidly adopted technology in civilization's history. As noted previously, the CDC has recognized that they must also reach adults who have only cell phones, and not just those with landlines, to gather complete data and, in turn, produce accurate reports. Likewise, other healthcare institutions must move to embrace mobile technologies so that they and the patients they serve have greater access to one another, and so that they can take advantage of the potential that these devices offer each of them for improved healthcare, greater efficiency, and lower costs. In general, there are two elements to these systems. One concerns the device itself, and the other is the way the device transmits and integrates information; that is, the network.

Categories of Wireless Technology and Networks

Wireless Local Area Networks and Wi-Fi

Wireless local area networks (WLANs) use spread-spectrum technology based on radio waves to enable devices in a limited area to communicate with one another within a range of 10 to 100 meters. This is what your local coffee shop or library may offer, and it is also the connectivity that a clinic or hospital may provide for users so that they can move around within its boundaries and still be connected. But connectivity beyond these boundaries is restricted. While the term *Wi-Fi* is considered by many to be synonymous with wireless Internet or WLAN, in a strict sense it refers only to products that are Wi-Fi certified based on the Institute of Electrical and Electronics Engineers (IEEE) 802.11 standards. IEEE is an international professional technical association that has developed over 1,000 standards addressing communication, electromagnetic compatibility, local and metropolitan area networks (LAN/MAN) standards, the family of 801 wireless standards, and portable application standards. Most personal computers (PCs), laptops, and smartphones, as well as peripherals, such as printers and fax machines, can operate within a WLAN. They also may be Wi-Fi certified. Health information managers should be aware that systems based on IEEE Wi-Fi standards 802.11a or 802.11b may not be sufficiently secure to meet healthcare documentation standards and may not be compliant with the Health Insurance Portability and Accountability Act (HIPAA) or the American Recovery and Reinvestment Act of 2009 (ARRA). Newer systems based on 802.11g and higher are preferred.

Each Wi-Fi station or access point may connect all wireless devices in that area with each other and with either the main information center or the Internet. Any healthcare provider may create a network of such Wi-Fi stations throughout the campus with special security for each Wi-Fi area. Most are created for institutional users, but such areas are also needed for visitors and are increasingly being offered in public areas such as registration or the coffee shop, reflecting a growing interest in addressing the needs and preferences of patients and visitors.

Wireless Wide-Area Networks

The term *cell phone* is derived from the use of a system of cell towers to connect early mobile phones. These cell towers enable wireless wide-area networks (WWANs) that allow users to transfer data electronically throughout the boundaries of the cellular network to which they subscribe. The boundaries may be regional, national, or even international, although at each level, limitations are likely, depending upon the cellular system offered by the user's telecommunications carrier (for example, Verizon, Sprint, AT&T, T-Mobile).

In the 1980s, these functions were described as "1G" (first generation). By the 1990s, 2G offered digitally encrypted conversations and data services, including text messages (short message service or SMS). Competition among the various regional and semiproprietary approaches increased the power of wireless computing. At about the same time, efforts to create a single, unified worldwide standard were ineffective, and several different standards were subsequently introduced.

Now most devices are based on 3G technology, a global standard for third generation wireless communications. These 3G devices meet a set of requirements (for example, data rates) and offer advanced mobile services that include not only voice but also image and data transmission, and they offer a range of functionalities that vary not only from device to device (for example, from basic voice phone to so called smartphones such as the iPhone, G1 Android, or latest Blackberry) but also from telecommunications carrier to telecommunications carrier. Further, even similar functionalities are packaged, displayed, and used in various ways, depending upon the device and carrier offering them. Eagerly anticipated 4G devices will expand upon and improve current services and functionalities.

3G Broadband

National telecommunications carriers and operators such as Verizon, AT&T, Sprint, and T-Mobile, offer 3G mobile broadband service; that is, wireless high-speed Internet access through a portable modem, telephone, or other device that enables mobile devices to be operational far beyond the limits of WLAN services, though coverage may vary from carrier to carrier. The combination of Wi-Fi access and broadband creates a patchwork of wireless communication that provides Internet access and cell phone technology as the user moves about, thus enabling the integration of wireless voice and data communication. Data communication through Internet capabilities (both broadband and Wi-Fi), on the other hand, offers the Voice over Internet Protocol (VoIP), transmitting voice (converted to data) through the Internet, just as its name implies. Thus, VoIP allows phone calls to be conducted from any place inside or outside a building or even in cars, trains, and planes (where sanctioned) as long as the Internet connection is good enough for this application. Some cities and metropolitan areas have created systems that fully integrate Wi-Fi and broadband options. As a result, a user has a very good connection at any place within that city. The challenge for many hospitals and clinics is that users want more and faster wireless Internet access to information inside and outside institutional walls. For data intensive service, Wi-Fi is preferred not only for cost reasons but also for its higher speed. The challenge to any provider institution is to cover the complete compound with good connectivity. For instance, if a hospital is spread over a wide geographic area, coverage must integrate broadband with Wi-Fi in order to provide good connectivity anywhere within the provider facilities.

Personal Area Networks

A personal area network (PAN) is a computer network that allows communication among computer devices in proximity to one's person. Also called WPAN (wireless PAN), it allows information technology (IT) devices within the range (approximately 10 meters) of an individual to interconnect. A clinician, for example, could connect his laptop, cell phone, and fax machine through a PAN, or his mDevice in his pocket with a Bluetooth device at his ear. Some make the distinction that PANs are for individuals and WPANs are local area networks (LANs) that connect multiple users wirelessly to multiple users (see WLAN and Wi-Fi discussed previously) (SearchMobileComputing.com, 2008). PANs may be wired with computer buses; that is, physical connections shared among multiple hardware components so they can communicate (for example, multiple-port USB drives). WPANs also can be enabled with network technologies such as Infrared Data Association (IrDA) standards that allow data transfer between devices without physical cables.

Data Communication and Security

Some readers may remember the rise of data communication in the form of the facsimile or fax. Today, the scanning of a document and then its transmission, generally known as faxing, is considered by many to be an outdated technology, although its use within healthcare persists, particularly in communications to and from physician practices that have not yet adopted EMRs. While the technical security of fax transmissions is, or at least can be, designed to meet HIPAA and ARRA regulations, some threats continue to warrant attention. For example, HIM professionals need to create systems and policies that assure that faxes are sent to the correct and authorized destination, and when received at that destination, the faxes are protected against exposure of private health information (PHI) to nonauthorized personnel. Secure data transmission also has been added to mobile phones, but concerns about authorized destination and receipt must still be addressed.

Over the last decade, the voice or telephone function has become just one of several functions, and certainly not the major one, that make mobile devices particularly valuable in many industries, including healthcare. This is because data communication has become more important than voice communication. As a result, the transmission of text is fast becoming a standard feature with new cell phones. Text transmission comes in many forms, including text messaging, e-mail, instant messaging, fax, and most recently, social media (for example, blogs, Twitter, and Facebook).

Text messaging or texting uses short message service (SMS) to send brief messages by cell phone. Indeed, brevity is required, as these text messages are restricted to 160 characters, including spaces. Most digital mobile phones and many personal digital assistants offer text messaging. People of all ages are embracing text messaging for easy, quick communication, with especially high adoption among young adults. The volume of text messaging demonstrates its appeal. In late December 2008, the *New York Times* reported "about 2.5 trillion messages will have been sent from cell phones worldwide this year" (Stross 2008).

Texting is not limited to cell phones. Increasingly, people are sending text conversations via their computers through systems such as Google or Yahoo. It is likely that you will encounter users who do not want to give up these communication methods when they work for your organization.

Initially, healthcare professionals avoided texting because it was viewed as insufficiently secure for healthcare applications, but some leading healthcare providers are adopting some very interesting text messaging applications because they recognize it as a preferred communication option for some patients.

Because such messages offer little security, text messaging should be mainly used for administrative messages such as appointment reminders or reminders to prepare for a test or to take medications. Nevertheless, some providers use it for brief clinical communications because it enables them to capture the attention of a patient who ignores or is otherwise unreachable through other forms of communications. Here's an example: "Nancy, u got a letter from Mem'l Clinic asking u 2 book an appt for a mammogram. To make an appt call 888-888-8888 today!" Text messages use brief forms, truncations, abbreviations, acronyms, and clipped sentences in order to stay within the 160-character limit. Several companies offer systems that allow the same message to be texted to thousands of patients. Thus, a provider can select a patient group and send all its members appropriate messages or reminders. For example, in the event of another medication recall such as that for Vioxx, a provider could text all her patients on the recalled medication to ask them to contact the office for an important message. For those preferring e-mail communications, the text message could tell them to check their e-mail as soon as possible for an important message. Those who prefer phone messages could be given a phone number to call, perhaps a number reserved for special messages, so that each caller hears the same message about the medication recall and what to do next. Perhaps some patients prefer instant messaging, which would allow real-time back and forth communication (discussed next). Of course, the use of text messaging to communicate clinical information should be authorized by the patient.

On many low-cost and older cell phones, texting is done with a numeric keyboard (the original telephone keyboard), requiring that users, for example, press the "6" key twice to type an *n* or the "7" key four times to type an *s*, and so forth. This is not acceptable to some older users, including clinicians, but younger people have learned the process quickly. That skill, together with specific text acronyms has captured the younger generation. Just as some health information professionals were trained in shorthand in the 1950s to 1970s, now some are learning today's electronic shorthand. Of course, in order to communicate most effectively with such patients, healthcare professionals must master the acronyms of texting and other electronic messages. Such acronyms and their meanings include 2nite (tonight), ADR (address), F2F (face-to-face), IAC (in any case), INPO (in no particular order), NRN (no reply necessary), OTOH (on the other hand) (Pinstack.com 2005). Given the widespread, notorious, and sometimes potentially dangerous use of abbreviations in healthcare, caution is called for in the use of "eAbbreviations" and "eAcronyms" in clinical communications that could confuse or mislead the reader.

Instant messaging can facilitate "live" communications with patients. It is real-time, synchronized text communication between two or more parties without the character limit of text messaging. This is in contrast to SMS, which is not necessarily either real time or synchronous; that is, the gap between sending and viewing a text message can be delayed anywhere from seconds to minutes, and a response, if any, may take place immediately after reading a text message or at some time later. Instant messaging is the equivalent of a phone conversation in that the messages pass back and forth in real time. Concerns for security are similar to those for text messages, and so, as with text messages, use of instant messaging for clinical communications should be authorized by the patient.

Faxing a message is another form of data transmission by cell phone. For instance, a patient may carry a copy of her personal health (PHR) record on her cell phone. To make sure that the physician knows about her medication list and her allergies, she sends these relevant parts of her personal health record to her provider prior to her appointment. If the provider does not have an EMR or other computer system to capture such information and enter it into the clinical information system, the information may be received as a printed fax.

Newer cell phones also offer e-mail, which can be an easy and convenient way to communicate safely and securely with the healthcare system because it can be encrypted. Since the early years of the 21st century, e-mail has slowly gained popularity as the preferred communication method between many patients and providers and among various caregivers, pharmacies, and health plans. Indeed, in some states, insurers reimburse providers for e-mail encounters, and over time, it is anticipated that this may be the case in all states. Though the reimbursement rate for an e-mail "visit" is considerably less than that for an office visit, providers embracing it recognize that e-mail encounters both take less time and free up valuable appointment slots for seeing patients who require an office visit. Again, it's important that patients agree to this form of communication, and that agreement generally includes an acknowledgement that e-mail will not be used for urgent or emergency situations and that the provider's response time may be as long as 24 to 48 hours. Many patients and providers prefer e-mail communications to telephone messaging, which oftentimes results in multiple voicemail messages or phone tag. Further, e-mail communications themselves create a documentation record, whereas telephone communications require an additional documentation process.

Even social networking is coming to healthcare. In a *New York Times* column, Dr. Pauline Chen discussed "Medicine in the age of Twitter." Social media can help coordinate care with both patients and specialists, assist in monitoring care, expand support networks, and strengthen the patient-doctor relationship. They can be especially useful in disease management, allowing communication to extend beyond office visits. Some physicians use blogs to provide education and to create connections and networks (Chen 2009).

Of course, these forms of text transmission require policies to address communication, technical, and medicolegal issues, in particular patient privacy. Back in 1998, Doctors Beverly Kane and Danny Sands coauthored the first guidelines for e-mail use in patient care. Given that their definition of e-mail was "Patient-provider electronic mail is defined as computer-based communication between clinicians and patients within a contractual relationship in which the health care provider has taken on an explicit measure of responsibility for the patient's care," you only need to substitute *communication* for *mail*, and it could also apply to the other forms of electronic communication described previously. Likewise, the policy considerations they recommend be addressed could be applied to other electronic communications, such as text messages and instant messaging:

- **Triage**—Who triages the communications and what is the response time?

- **Clerical overhead**—How will messages be integrated into patients' medical records?

- **Categorization and redirection**—Should electronic communications be categorized by provider, each with its own account, or by category (for example, billing, clinical, scheduling), or by both provider and category?

- **Selective access to providers**—Will the provider's electronic address be released to all patients or selectively?

- **Archiving and backup**—Whose server should be used for archiving and backup—the provider's, the institution's, or both? Also, who should schedule archiving, clearing, and indexing for storage and retrieval?

- **Forbidden topics**—Should highly sensitive topics such as HIV and behavioral conditions be allowed or disallowed?

- **Selective confidentiality**—Can patients opt to exclude certain electronic communication content from their records, and if so, is a secure repository required for such exclusions? Do state laws allow such exclusions and archiving?

- **Encryption**—Should all communications be encrypted or only those with clinical content? How is that determined and by whom?

- **Clinic-provided e-mail accounts**—Will patients be offered e-mail accounts (or instant message or blogs) on the facility's server? Inside or outside the firewall?

- **Outcomes evaluation**—What factors will be used to evaluate efficacy and usefulness—Cost-benefit analysis, patient satisfaction, provider satisfaction, clinical outcomes?

More recently, Dr. Scott Albin (2009) drafted basic guidelines for doctors on Facebook that include, for example, not requiring patients to participate, not "friending" patients, and never giving medical advice on Facebook.

Images and Security

Most cell phones these days have a built-in camera. The quality of photos taken by these cameras has improved so much that some users no longer have or use a traditional digital or analog camera. The mDevice allows not only easy picture-taking but also the swift transmission of such pictures to others, as well as quick and easy storage and organization of images. The use of an mDevice as a camera means that patients can take pictures of wounds, rashes, or injuries and send them as e-mail attachments to their provider for assessment. Similarly, changes over time can be photographed and forwarded to facilitate ongoing assessment and continuous recordkeeping, without repeat (and costly) office visits.

Clinicians also can receive photos and other clinical images, such as x-rays and EKG readings, on their cell phones for initial assessment if they do not have immediate access to such images on a PC or laptop. In third world countries, cell phones transmit images that would otherwise not be accessible. Some cell phones offer not only still pictures but also video recording, allowing, for example, a clinician to assess the gait of an injured patient. In recent years, some behavioral clinics have experimented with taking admission and exit videos, some of which are taken with mDevices. New guidelines and policies are needed to bring such videos into the health information system.

The full potential of the use of these cell phone cameras in the clinical environment has not yet been thoroughly explored or assessed, and it must be acknowledged that videos and still images may pose a threat to confidentiality. Imagine the consequences if a technician took video of the mammogram of a famous politician or the hernia exam of the local mayor. Some clinics and hospitals may go so far as to restrict healthcare professionals (and visitors) from using mDevices with cameras or requiring that the cameras in such devices be disabled. However, institutions may find it difficult to enforce such restrictions. Thus, education and guidelines regarding appropriate use of such devices are critical, as is information regarding the consequences of such misuse.

Internet Resources

The centuries-long dream of a "thinking machine" began to be realized for the masses with the introduction of the personal computer in the 1970s. Laptops, first introduced in the 1980s, gained popularity and capacity as they became more powerful but smaller and lighter. Today, many clinicians routinely carry mDevices such as smartphones, laptops or tablets during hospital rounds, preferring them to paper records because they offer easy, real-time, point-of-care access capture and transmission of patient and other information, including Internet resources.

Indeed, the biggest change in our society over recent decades is the Internet, and it continues to evolve and to offer connectivity and access to information in ways that were unimaginable just a few years ago. The Internet is a huge, self-correcting, and rapidly expanding source of information. If you Google "health," you will find more than one million pages of entries about health on the Internet. Certainly, there is no question that it holds and offers access to much more information than any person can memorize or has ever before had direct, real-time access to, and with mDevices, that access is available anywhere, anytime, to anyone.

That is the power of mDevices, particularly in healthcare: Internet searches no longer require access to PCs or laptops. Cell phones with browsers allow clinicians to access information in the exam room and while on the go, indeed anywhere, anytime. This opens up a whole new and expanding world of healthcare information as caregivers can instantly, and without regard to location, look up almost any topic within the scientific body of medicine. In other words, the mobile device in a clinician's hand provides him with the power of the Internet and enables him to access information from sources around the globe. For instance, when a patient doesn't remember the name of the medication she is taking but can describe it or has a sample with her, the nurse can identify the pill on his mDevice and doesn't have to resort to print resources that are incomplete and out of date upon publication. Systems providing such services are currently available at very low prices on the iPhone, for example.

Similarly, the Internet helps patients and others to access information about symptoms, medications, and any other health issue or concern. With the cell phone, a patient can look up a medication that was just prescribed by his clinician and learn more about its side effects and how it should be taken. He might, for example, note that the medication interacts negatively with another medication he is taking but that he neglected to tell his physician about, whether that lapse was intentional or not.

As we approach the end of the 21st century's first decade, the Internet is a de facto second opinion to numerous patients and healthy people. The Pew Internet Project reports, "83 percent of internet users, or 61 percent of U.S. adults" have looked online for health information" (Fox 2009). The Internet is also a tremendous resource for clinicians. Initially, there was substantial concern within the medical community about the value of the information that the Internet offered, with many believing that Internet information might be harmful to patients because some of it is unauthorized. These concerns have diminished as the power of self-correction and quick identification of false information has been recognized. Additionally, search engine techniques reduce the likelihood of accessing misleading or harmful information because the most reliable and most often requested information is generally displayed with more prominence. Further, a Health on the Internet Code of Content (HONcode) was developed to stimulate both Web site developers to meet basic ethical standards and consumers to seek the source and purpose of the information they read on the Internet. Briefly, the eight principles of HON content are: authoritative, complementarity (that is, supporting patient-physician relationship), privacy, attribution, justifiability, transparency, financial disclosure, and advertising policy. Certified sites display the HON Foundation symbol and are considered trustworthy. However, it must be acknowledged that adoption of the HONcode is not yet widespread (Health on the Internet Foundation 2008).

The level of acceptance of the validity of information available through the Internet has increased substantially over the last 10 years. Still, many professionals remain skeptical. In any case, both patients and healthcare professionals researching the Web for health- and disease-related information are well advised to seek such information from recognized and trusted sites. The National Institutes of Health has extensive resources, as do such major medical centers as Johns Hopkins and the Mayo Clinic. Widely recognized Web-only sites include WebMD and Medline. Other important resources include disease-specific organizations such as the American Heart Association, the National Multiple Sclerosis Society, and the Alzheimer's Association. Further, it is important for patients to discuss their research with their providers, particularly when it conflicts with or supplements what their clinician has communicated to them.

Through application service provider (ASP) services empowered by the browser, providers and patients can run many healthcare applications on their cell phones. ASP businesses provide their customers with Internet-based computing capabilities that transform the cell phone into a hand-held, lightweight, portable computer; that is, into a handheld device that is not only smaller, lighter, and easier to handle than a PC or laptop but that also has increased computing power that exceeds that of some PCs and laptops. Today, many patients and physicians are finding that it is easier, faster, and more convenient to access a Web site over a smartphone than to use their desktop computer. Until just a few years ago, such mDevices were called personal digital assistants (PDAs). From the 1980s to the 1990s, their popularity exploded due to a number of extended memory and notebook functions. Initially promoted and viewed as handheld computers, PDAs have evolved to offer voice as well as computer services, and today they are more likely to be called smartphones. Some of these smartphones have built-in small keyboards, others have touch screen keyboards, and some offer both keyboard types.

mDevices also can be used as speech recorders, transforming them into note takers or dictation devices for medical transcription and other purposes. Supplemented with speech recognition technology, the mDevice can facilitate real-time speech-to-text documentation. These voice functions on some devices also allow the user to make phone calls by speaking the name or number of the party to be called rather than by entering it manually.

Another interesting use of voice with mobile devices is voice badges. These lightweight badges are clipped to a person's clothing, and combined with speech recognition, they route calls automatically, connecting the user with the emergency team she needs or the admitting office, for example, without having to open either a wireless or a manual directory (Davis 2004).

Selecting Devices

All cell phones are not equal. To be attractive to buyers, cell phone manufacturers develop phones with specific capabilities tailored for a specific market. Thus, types of cell phones or mDevices include all-around mobile phones, luxury and designer phones, photo or camera phones, music phones, multimedia phones, navigation phones, touch screen phones, PDAs, Web phones, Web radio devices and phones, notebooks, subnotebooks, tablets, laptops, wireless medical devices, and so on. These names are meant to be descriptive yet nonlimiting. For example, navigation phones have their strength in GPS navigation but are likely to offer a number of other functions.

HIM professionals, chief information officers (CIOs), and others have long been asking, "Shouldn't we select a specific cell phone device for all our clinicians and employees in order to standardize mDevice adoption in our organization?" or "What mobile device should we require our clinicians to use?" The response to these questions may reflect the culture of an organization, but organizations should consider a strategy that allows users to select their own devices because "one size does not fit all," and since many clinicians see patients in two or more provider institutions, they will not react enthusiastically if they are required to use a different device in each institution.

Personal preferences will vary. For some, size and weight may be the most important consideration. For example, users may not like the small screen and the small keyboard of smartphones. Other users may not like the heavier weight of tablets or laptops. Some like the touch screen of iPhones and similar devices, while others prefer a keyboard. Regarding keyboards, some may insist on a QWERTY layout, while others may be more comfortable with phone key pads, where multiple taps on number keys result in letter entry.

But keyboards and phone key pads speak only to the "touch and feel factor" of mDevices. The software associated with different mDevices on different platforms can vary tremendously. At present, the iPhone is the absolute leader in volume and variety of healthcare-related software, offering more than 5,000 healthcare-related applications and thousands of other applications. On the other hand, if security is an issue, products from Research in Motion (RIM), such as the Blackberry, are currently (in 2010) considered by many to be most secure. However, it is important to keep in mind that such assessments can change quickly because the industry is rapidly evolving and new features and services are offered almost daily in this exploding market.

This means that healthcare organizations that do not select and provide the same device to all their users must develop policies that can accommodate a range of mDevices. Some hospitals and clinics may offer users the option of selecting devices that best suit the user but that at the same time fit into the organizational strategy regarding functionality, security, integration, and interoperability. (See Chapter 4 for additional guidance on selecting mDevices, as well as mApplications.)

The Role of mDevices in Healthcare

As described above, cell phones are the most widely adopted and successful new technology device in history. Many users, in particular young people, will not leave home without their cell phone, giving it the same importance as keys or a wallet. Further, the cell phone is on its way to becoming a digital companion that can do much more than just communicate with others. Calendar functions, note-taking, and similar secretarial functions are common, along with the previously mentioned camera functions. Geographic intelligence systems are now being added to most advanced phones, giving directions and helping users find their way with their mDevices. Banking applications, music applications, and Web access through mDevices are changing our lives forever and will increasingly impact healthcare systems as well. Some cell phones, for example, can be used for such diverse functions as a flashlight, an alarm clock, a yoga instructor, or a financial transaction device at the same time that that they are also music players and cameras.

Cell phones also can be identification devices. In 2008, some airlines began allowing the cell phone to function as a boarding pass. Systems like "remember me" allow a cell phone user to register her identification with an airline, which then responds to every call from that phone with a personal greeting and immediate access to that person's reservations and other stored data. This identification method in healthcare would require that a patient register her phone as the communication identification medium for specific patient information and authorize the exchange of personal health information via this phone.

Alternatively, the phone may translate a telephone number into a specific bar code that can be linked to the patient's medical record number and that bar code could be scanned for identification when the individual shows up in person. Such identification systems are already used by a number of airlines. In general, HIM professionals are facing new ways of establishing identification. In addition to identifying the person who comes to the office, they also need to identify the person who is authorized to receive or send information from an mDevice. It may be the patient himself or it may be the patient's mother because she is most likely the family health manager, who will authorize communication on behalf of the entire family (with authorization, of course, in the case of family members who are adults). Keep in mind that specific attention must be given to information elements that are excluded from such authorizations.

In Europe, cell phones can be used to take public transportation or to purchase goods. "Money" is loaded onto the phone, thereby replacing cash. It is not out of the realm of possibility that the cell phone will become the digital companion that a person uses for numerous daily functions. It may become the one item that replaces your watch, keys, wallet, and even credit card and holds your Internet identification, personal health record, driver's license, passport, and access to online libraries, bank information, professional resources, and GPS for navigation. It may take another 5 to 10 years, or perhaps only 2 to 3, until we reach this point, but all indicators show that we are well on the way.

These likely possibilities will be welcomed by many, but the usual pushback and fear that new devices inevitably stimulate must be acknowledged. History books tell us, for example, that the stethoscope was initially ridiculed and that its acceptance took a long time. Likewise, the fear that cell phones cause cancer has not fully abated, although the National Cancer Institute reported in 2008 that cell phones are safe (Wenner 2008). Still, many await longer-term studies to prove or disprove this concern.

What is mHealth?

Mobile health, also known as mHealth, is a new phenomenon that includes and far surpasses telemedicine and telehealth. It is also distinct from, although to a degree overlapping with, eHealth (see figure 1.1). mHealth encompasses all mobile, wireless technologies, systems, devices, and applications used to enable better communication in and delivery of healthcare. At its core is the ability to communicate by text, e-mail, image, and voice in combination with access to the Internet and computing capabilities. mHealth recognizes all cell phones, smartphones, PDAs, tablets, laptops, and other portable computing and communication devices as mobile devices (mDevices) and through these devices enables communication by all participating health stakeholders. In regards to public health, mHealth offers the opportunity to conduct greater health surveillance and reporting through participatory systems and facilitates instant notification of populations in case of a public health threat or emergency.

mHealth has different applications in various parts of the world. Countries in North America, Europe, and other areas, which have advanced health information systems but are held back by legacy systems, are creating new communication patterns enabled by mHealth. Countries, such as Brazil and India, that are not limited by the technological experiences of other countries or by their legacy systems are using mHealth to leapfrog health information technology and to enable new technologies for efficient electronic care (eCare). Some less developed countries (for example, some nations in Africa and Asia) that

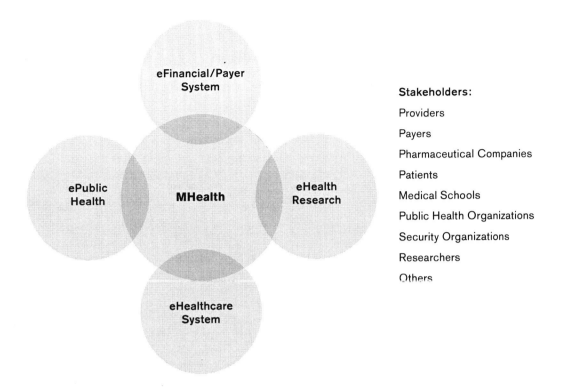

Stakeholders:

Providers

Payers

Pharmaceutical Companies

Patients

Medical Schools

Public Health Organizations

Security Organizations

Researchers

Others

Figure 1.1   Overlapping eHealth and mHealth

are infrastructure-challenged, are adopting very basic uses of cell phones in healthcare with sometimes remarkable results, including SMS-directed emergency surgery and public health disease monitoring to a degree previously impossible and unimaginable. Additionally, basic voice communication through mDevices provides medical assistance that would otherwise be inaccessible in some areas.

EHRs, EMRs, PHRs, and Interoperability

Healthcare visionaries have long recognized the value of a healthcare system that provides all the relevant information that a caregiver needs at the point of care, but efforts needed to achieve this seem overwhelming. In the early 1990s, the Institute of Medicine offered what appeared to be the solution: a longitudinal electronic health record (EHR) system that would connect a patient's data from all the hospitals, clinics, or other places where she had received services over her lifetime. Hopes for achieving such a system in the anticipated 10-year time frame were quickly shattered, and the achievement of a universally interoperable EHR system that has uniform documentation remains in the far distant future.

Meanwhile providers continue to struggle with what evolved into a more limited vision; that is, the EMR that allows the electronic collection and maintenance of patient data within a single healthcare enterprise. The slow adoption of EMRs is due, at least in part, to the fact that it shifts the burden of documentation (if it is to be real time) mostly to the clinician, potentially eliminating transcription and its accompanying editing, which delay its completion and its ability to be shared. Thus, it takes the clinician longer to complete documentation, and it is more cumbersome and costly (at least in the short run) than paper-based documentation or even electronic transcription and editing as we know it today; further, there may be decreased accuracy due to lack of review by the clinician of both his own entries and those auto-filled by the mHealth application he uses. According to a *New England Journal of Medicine* national survey, fewer than 20 percent of providers nationwide reported having some form of an EMR and fewer than 5 percent reported having a fully functioning EMR (DesRoches 2008). Further, the lack of true interoperability, not only across disparate enterprises but sometimes even across departments within a single enterprise, frustrates the providers (and patients) and diminishes the value of electronic data, in turn limiting its positive impact.

For patients, this means that they cannot expect their doctor to know in a timely manner, if at all, what the specialist they saw recently described or prescribed or anything else that happened outside that provider's setting. They cannot routinely expect their records to be electronic or their providers to be linked to other providers and therefore be informed about their care across settings or even sometimes across departments within a clinic or hospital. In response, some patients have started to manage their own health data set in form of a personal health record (PHR). The objective of PHRs is not only to make such information available to the patient himself but also, at the person's discretion, to make it available to health practitioners (including personal physicians and pharmacists) across settings. For a time, smart cards, CDs, or USB sticks were used as the portable storage medium for PHRs, but clinicians and provider institutions rejected them for fear of the viruses that they may carry. In the not so distant future, cell phones are anticipated to be the medium of choice to communicate PHR information between patients and providers as they offer easier interoperability, not only because, unlike most EMRs, cell phones can communicate with one another, but also because most of today's PHRs are based on a standard composite data set—the Continuity of Care Record (CCR)—which is World Wide Web Consortium (W3C) XML-based, facilitating information exchange. (XML is a system designed to transport and store data.) Thus, HIM professionals are advised to prepare for PHR communications through mDevices. This means they must consider how their organization is prepared to receive and integrate the PHR information that patients send via their cell phone before the visit, and they must design systems to integrate such data automatically into the paper or EMR system and to update the CCR at the end of the visit to send back to the patient. The "PHR on the phone" will challenge traditional HIM practices. For more about the PHR on mobile devices, see Chapter 3.

The New Paradigm: Health Communications

A century ago, a patient would see his physician only when the injury or illness justified the expense and time required to do so. There was no continuous care, no preventive care, and no reason to see a physician except to take care of some severe symptoms or injury. Now, patients are encouraged to see their caregiver on a regular basis and to consider health maintenance as well as preventive screenings and care. Nevertheless, health communication is still at the level of the past century so that when a patient sees her clinician, she still must try to remember and communicate everything within the 10- to 15-minute window of the typical visit. mHealth has the potential to change this by providing systems that allow continuous communication between the patient and the clinician. Disease management programs and other care delivery enhancements are facilitated and enhanced through easy, accessible mDevice communication. In addition, mDevices offer the capacity to e-mail or text message requests for appointments, including the patient's agenda or reasons for a visit, and to receive instructions for tests to be done prior to a face-to-face visit. In general terms, patients will be able to stay in touch with their providers through mDevices and receive continuous care as needed. Such communication is only made possible through the new cell phone culture and the ability of mDevices to offer safe and secure communication from any place at any time.

Participatory Health

Another major movement, democratization of healthcare, is underway as we approach the second decade of the 21st century. The healthcare system is becoming more transparent, and care information is now available not only between clinicians and researchers but also between patients and others. Healthcare is being transformed from a clinician- and researcher-centric system into one that seeks to coordinate the roles of all healthcare participants, including patients. This new paradigm called participatory health, embraces patients, healthcare providers, wellness providers, payers, researchers, pharmacists, public health officials, and others as active and equal participants. mDevices and mHealth are its major enablers. Indeed, participatory health could not be implemented without mHealth and the Internet.

Influenced by mHealth developments and the democratization of healthcare, the movement toward participatory health has gathered historic strength. It is the shift away from "doctor as God" and toward the patient as the center of the healthcare system. Some experts see this as creating a transition from treatment in the clinic, doctor's office, or hospital to treatment in the home. However, participatory care goes much further. In participatory health, the focus is on communication between all the participants, including clinicians, health coaches, payers, pharmacists, and, of course, the patient herself. Such a system, with the patient at its center, could not be established and maintained without the voice, data, and Internet communication capabilities of mHealth. Truly, participatory health cannot fully blossom without mHealth and the communication capabilities that it offers. In turn, the full potential and impact of mHealth will be compromised without this movement toward participatory health.

mCare

A new approach to healthcare, called mCare is emerging. While mHealth begins by focusing on new ways for patients, clinicians, public health officials, and many others to communicate, exchange knowledge, and document at any location, mCare is that portion of it that relates specifically to the care process. It emphasizes care based on communication between patient and provider, especially through the connectivity of mDevices. The clinician may be located in another state or even in another country, but the care is expected to be better and more continuous if the patient and clinician exchange observations and correspond on health issues and disease conditions than if the care is based on sporadic patient visits for acute conditions or chronic care checkups and flare-ups.

mCare involves:

- Patients and providers communicating continuously
- Reducing face-to-face visits to a minimum
- Clinicians and patients actively and in tandem researching the scientific body of medicine via the Web as a routine part of the care process
- Collecting increasing amounts of data from mDevices and wirelessly integrating them into the care process
- Exchanging still images and video (patients sending pictures or videos of their health/disease condition, clinicians sending videos of patient education)
- Conducting administrative functions, such as registration in a hospital and determining insurance eligibility, in a virtual mode between provider and patient
- Involving authorized others (for example, spouses, parents of younger patients, children of elderly patients) in the care process
- Synchronizing a patient-controlled PHR with the data that providers keep
- Integrating medical care with behavioral care and concerns of well being

In summary, mHealth has many facets and components, including devices, applications, mCare, participatory health, regional emphases, institutional designs, and personalized care plans. All of these components are based on enhanced communication that is aimed at improving care, whether for individuals or a population and whether in a single provider setting, city, country, or worldwide.

mHealth's Application Clusters

Introduction

The pace at which patients, consumers, clinicians and other healthcare providers, payers, public health professionals, researchers, and others are adopting and using cell phones and other mDevices is fueling the development of mHealth applications. The biggest growth in applications in 2009 were on the iPhone. Apple provided a simple application for users to create their own software, and more than 1,000 users have developed over 100,000 iPhone applets, of which over 2,000 are health related. But mHealth applications extend far beyond that one system's approach. iPhone competitors include the Android G1, the Blackberry, and others, which have several hundred healthcare applications. The range and pace of new applications is overwhelming, but even more impressive is their impact on healthcare and healthcare delivery. We will explore these applications through a review of the 12 mHealth application clusters into which the mHealth Initiative has categorized them (see Figure 2.1) (Waegemann 2009a).

Application Cluster 1: Patient Communication

The mHealth revolution has a complex system of patient communication at its core that includes communications before, during, and after a visit to the healthcare provider, as well as nonvisit-related communications.

Communication between Patients and Providers

As noted earlier, patients traditionally saw their physicians only when needed and often not for months or years at a time. In response to the recognition that health maintenance requires different care patterns than illness care, patients now are

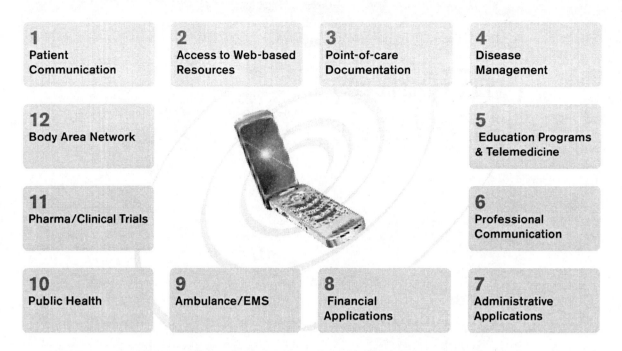

1
Patient
Communication

2
Access to Web-based
Resources

3
Point-of-care
Documentation

4
Disease
Management

12
Body Area Network

5
Education Programs
& Telemedicine

11
Pharma/Clinical Trials

6
Professional
Communication

10
Public Health

9
Ambulance/EMS

8
Financial
Applications

7
Administrative
Applications

FIGURE 2.1   12 mobile phone application clusters in healthcare

encouraged to see their clinicians on a more regular basis for routine and preventive check-ups and tests. Nevertheless, these visits still tend to be infrequent and brief and only selective health and wellness concerns are being addressed. And with diminishing numbers of primary care physicians, the demand and need for care will increasingly exceed the supply of both physicians and time. Thus, the healthcare field is at a crossroads. When is it really necessary to be with the clinician? Could most of the patient-provider exchange at a visit be communicated online? Would such offline communications enable more continuous and effective intervention at lower costs? Should office visits be reserved for care that requires face-to-face interaction? These questions are among those being discussed as we face a major restructuring of our healthcare system. But the questioning of face-to-face visits goes even further. Are there situations where an office visit is at best useless or at worst misleading or harmful? For example, think of a child with asthma being evaluated in the clinician's office when electronically sending data generated in her normal home and school environments would provide more valuable information.

mHealth offers expanding communication opportunities between patients and providers, communication that will fill the gap between physical encounters according to patients' and/or providers' needs. The use of mDevices by consumers and healthcare professionals enables them to change the pattern of occasional or sporadic physician/patient encounters to a system of continuous communication that enhances healthcare and wellness, while reducing costly visits. And this can be done without placing an additional burden on the provider. The goal of mHealth is to create a health ecosystem that facilitates communication across the spectrum of healthcare stakeholders—patients/consumers, healthcare providers, wellness providers, and others.

There are five requisites to achieving this vision of mHealth:

1. A provider organization must facilitate cell phone use throughout its facility, taking appropriate measures to assure electromagnetic compatibility. Health information management professionals have a unique opportunity to influence decision making related to allowing patients, clinicians, and others to use modern communication systems to support maximum quality of care.

2. Patients must be stimulated to have regular communications with their providers.

3. In turn, providers must accept changes in workflow and systems in order to make such communication both time-saving and productive.

4. Payers must revise reimbursement systems to include adequate payments that support this new system of communication.

5. Appropriate security and confidentiality policies and guidelines must be designed and implemented.

The degree to which patients and the general public adopt new communication patterns (for example, e-mail and text messaging) as forms of healthcare communication varies depending upon their familiarity and comfort level with these modes. Physicians and other health professionals who have completed education and training within the past few years are mDevice "natives." Within the general population, those from early childhood (even as young as age 4) to 30 or 35 are already familiar with this new technology and are embracing this new opportunity to use these familiar and preferred communication methods. Others who are a bit older and who are at least e-mail and cell phone savvy, recognize fairly quickly that these technologies can improve their own health and the health of their children and older family members for whom they are responsible.

For those who are unfamiliar with or resistant to new technologies, persuasive education campaigns are necessary. And for some, device and application design eases them toward adoption. Specially designed phones that are simple to use are more attractive to some seniors than are the latest gadgets with lots of bells and whistles (Waegemann 2009b).

In order for the mHealth communication systems to achieve maximum benefits, substantial changes must be made at the organizational level. HIM professionals, for example, can play a key role in designing and delivering educational campaigns to patients and other consumers, just as they are already involved in encouraging patients to adopt personal health records (PHRs).

PHRs are important tools to create interoperability between providers. For instance, your enterprise may have succeeded in having all patient information from various departments and satellite sites combined into a centralized electronic medical record; if so, this is the exception. To maximize the quality of healthcare delivery, providers must have access to relevant information on care delivered not only by a particular institution but also that provided in nonaffiliated settings. Think of a patient who recently went to a specialist without referral from the clinicians in your organization. In such cases, the PHR with its CCR-based core data set is the potential tool of interoperability that enables continuity of care. These PHRs are an important component in efforts to increase communication between patients and providers through the use of mDevices.

In 2003, AHIMA acknowledged the importance of PHRs when it created the MyPHR Web site (www.myphr.com) to promote and educate the public about the PHR and to provide guidance on how to create one (AHIMA e-HIM Personal Health Record Work Group 2005). Further, since November 2008, it has trained more than 1,500 HIM professionals on how to speak and educate the public on the PHR; as of September 2009 more than 600 additional HIM professionals had been trained (AHIMA, 2008; May 2009).

The PHR is a tremendous opportunity for HIM professionals in other ways as well. Templates for structured communication must be designed and implemented. Incoming text messages and e-mails must be managed according to their importance and urgency. HIM professionals are prime candidates to manage the stream of patient communication and process those e-mails and messages that do not need clinician attention, while bringing critical and urgent messages to clinicians' attention immediately. Policies and procedures must be developed that enable clinicians to read and process the less important messages in the least time-consuming and most efficient way. Perhaps a new role and title for HIM professionals is evolving—the health information communication manager. For more information on the PHR, see Chapter 3.

Patient Communications: New Patterns and Security Considerations

Information management professionals are already being asked to develop electronic communication (eCommunication patterns). Some rules apply:

First, a good identification system is essential. Some providers might offer a cell phone identification system that recognizes a person calling from a registered phone. Imagine that the mother is the family's health manager coordinating all her family members' appointments and health issues. Following her enrollment in, and authorization of, such a system, when she calls in, the phone system will recognize her and greet her, "Hello, Mrs. Williams, thank you for calling Dr. Johnson's office. We have been authorized to allow you to address all four members of your family. About whom are you calling today?" The identification system then can be linked to the EMR system, and when Mrs. Williams has communicated that she is calling about her daughter Sarah, the system automatically notes "Sarah is due for a refill of her medication. Is this what you are calling about, or do you want to schedule an appointment?"

Unless otherwise authorized, text messaging should be used only for administrative communication such as appointment management and reminders of tests. And again, advance authorization by the patient for its use must be documented. Where options for reminder systems (telephone, e-mail, text messaging) are offered, more patients are electing text messaging as the simplest, easiest, most direct form of reminder. Depending on the institutional policy and state regulations, these administrative messages may or may not be kept in the patient's medical record or in a separate administrative file. It is important to note, too, that such electronic reminders are less costly than postcard or letter reminders and are less time consuming than phone reminders.

Of course, all clinical communication should be secured with encryption. In most cases, secure e-mail is used for clinical communications such as responses to patient's inquiries about something they researched on the Internet, their symptoms or other health matters. Even when the patient's inquiry comes in the form of a text message, secure e-mail is the preferred response medium, unless, of course, the patient has requested and authorized text messages regarding clinical matters.

Most commercial e-mail systems are not secure. Thus, providers have created secure e-mail systems that are contained within their Web portal or their virtual private network (VPN). Most of these systems are not very user-friendly and require patients to go through a cumbersome process to log in and communicate with their provider by e-mail. This is changing, and new encryption-based commercial e-mail systems are expected to be available in early 2010 that will provide "clinical grade email"; that is, e-mail that is safe, secure, and confidential, and is as easy and intuitive as the most popular e-mail systems. In any case, such clinical communications with patients should always be considered part of the medical record.

Most cell phones these days routinely offer camera functions, and special attention should be paid to restrictions against caregivers, employees, contractors, or other institutional personnel taking photos or videos that are not clinically justified. Photos that are taken for clinical purposes must be included in the patient's medical record.

Previsit Communications

mDevices facilitate advance communication before any physical encounter between a patient and a provider and may help determine that such a visit is not necessary or should be delayed until further information, such as lab data, is available. This preparatory process encourages patients at the time they inquire about an appointment to submit a structured communication template (designed and generated by the provider institution) to send their personal health data, including their insurance eligibility information from their mDevice to their provider. This template enables the patient to state in appropriate detail the reason for the visit, giving providers the opportunity to prepare for the visit, including, for example, ordering tests to be done in advance of a visit rather than following it. They may also consult resources to supplement their knowledge about signs and.symptoms and thus prepare for the visit or for nonvisit intervention. Such a template allows the patient to reference Internet-researched information that they want to discuss. This new process can reduce the number of follow-up visits and enable implementation of a more-informed plan of care.

Such previsit components require educational campaigns for patients as well as clinicians, particularly regarding necessary workflow changes. They also may stimulate means of reimbursement for eCommunication and for pre-encounter preparations that could reduce the time necessary for a visit or even replace a visit. So, again, these are opportunities for HIM professionals to enhance their role in the institution by helping to design and deliver such educational campaigns and by working with financial officers to assure that the documentation for eCommunication reimbursement is adequate and timely.

Communications during an Episode of Care

Providers and patients are beginning to use eCommunication on a continuing basis. Rather than limiting communications to the short time of an encounter, patients and providers stay in regular electronic communication. While e-mail communications are already commonly used, some providers are experimenting with text messaging. Such increased communication could lead to a reduction in the number of visits required and in greater continuity of care. As noted above, this will require revisions in reimbursement systems to allow payments for e-mails and text messages (where these are not already reimbursed) in order to make this new mode of communication more attractive for providers. Such increased communication between patients and providers could reduce office visits by as much as 20 percent (Waegemann 2009b). In addition, disease management supported by digital communications is demonstrating great success as described later in this chapter.

General Follow-up and Other Communications

The goals of improved patient satisfaction and enhanced competitiveness are also among the factors driving providers toward new communication methods. A system that can send out automatic text messages the day after a visit has great potential. A simple text message such as, "How r u?" from the physician that stimulates a timely response of "Fine" or "Not so good" can indicate whether a follow-up appointment or some other intervention is indicated, at the same time that it reassures the patient that the physician is concerned about his care.

Post-surgical patients can use mDevices to easily communicate their recovery experiences, keeping their provider aware of routine recovery experiences but also quickly alerting him when unexpected signs and symptoms occur. Some of these reports are automatically sent from monitoring devices through the cell phone to the provider. Additionally, post-surgical patients are using mDevices to access online patient forums to communicate with other patients who have experienced similar surgeries in order to compare post-op experiences.

Enhanced communication also can lead to better compliance rates. Some mDevice applications remind the patient of medications, appointments, and tests, and more applications are in development.

The use of telecommunication systems that connect the provider and the patient's home is expanding. As such systems are integrated into the participatory health process, patients and providers can be linked electronically, medications monitored, and signs and symptoms checked remotely. A wide range of such applications are being implemented for home care, and numerous others are under development.

Connectivity between existing home monitoring systems and mDevices allows communication and monitoring throughout the patient's living space, including alerts to falls or other accidents. Data collection and transmission to the main monitoring system is part of the design of these systems, and in-home displays are being expanded from mDevices to TV, computer, and display units.

Advantages of mDevice monitoring include that routine data can be easily and quickly collected and communicated to the provider with little effort on the part of the patient. In turn, patients are easily reminded to take medications, check blood sugar, keep appointments, and comply with guidelines. With the mDevice continuously available, emergency calls can be made directly from the device. Additionally, fencing applications are available that monitor the whereabouts of an Alzheimer patient, for example, thus preventing incidents of the patient wandering off.

Connectivity between medical devices and information systems, including mHealth, must be made more secure to ensure minimum standards of quality of service (QoS). Several organizations, including Continua, the Food and Drug Administration (FDA), the Joint Commission, and IEEE, are addressing issues of interoperability, potential electromagnetic interference (EMI), data integrity, and security. These are key issues for HIM professionals to be alert to as we enter the era of mHealth.

In summary, traditional patient communications are being replaced by new communication patterns. Table 2.1 contrasts the old and new communications methods and summarizes their impact on HIM.

Application Cluster 2: Access to Web-based Resources

The power of the Internet on the mDevice is tremendous. It has opened up a whole new world of information covering all scholarly disciplines as well as every aspect of everyday life. Geographic positioning systems (GPS) can find anyone's location and provide directions from there to where they wish to go and back. Consider any aspect of science, commerce, or communication, and you'll find thousands, of online resources.

TABLE 2.1 Traditional and new communication methods between patients and healthcare providers and their impact on HIM

Traditional Patient Communication Systems	New Patient Communication Systems	Impact on HIM
Patient communicates with clinician on an "as needed" basis	Continuous communication for preventive purposes, disease management, healthier lifestyle, etc. Provider communication urges compliance/cooperation.	New systems must be created and managed to accommodate 24/7 communication and related documentation.
Patient and clinician communicate mainly in face-to-face visits	Patient communicates electronically by voice, data, images.	Confidentiality must be assured in all modes of communication.
Little or no pre-visit communication. Patients tell provider at visit the reason for visit.	Patients sends agenda (reason for visit) in advance. Provider may offer instructions before visit.	New opportunities to educate and monitor patients. Systems must accommodate documentation.
Beginning of home monitoring.	More communication with the patient through monitors connected to their cell phones, TV, body area networks, etc.	Must select and monitor new systems for user friendliness, data integrity, authentication, and confidentiality.
Occasional wireless communication between medical devices and the HIT system	Mainly wireless communication between medical devices and the HIT system.	Must assure data integrity, EMC, authentication, quality of service, permanence, confidentiality.
Physician accesses patient information from paper record or electronic medical record	Patient information is accessed from mDevices, EMR, the personal health record, etc.	Coordination and synchronization is needed.
Patient communicates only general, occasional, or summary information. Few details.	Observations of Daily Living (ODLs) give precise patient observations.	Specific systems must be created to capture, manage, and integrate ODLs into the patient's records.

According to a 2009 Pew research report, "74% of American adults go online, 57% of American households have broadband connections, and 61% of adults look online for health information." The report calls these users "e-patients" and further notes that 'always present' mobile access draws people into conversations about health as much as online tools enable research" (Fox 2009). Their report includes these observations:

- American adults integrate both traditional sources of health information with their increasing use of online tools
- the majority of e-patients seek user-generated health-related information, that is, from someone just like themselves, although there is limited use of social networking sites for such information
- online research impacts their health decisions, with more positive than negative experiences being reported
- Internet health-related research extends to exercise and fitness
- change is coming whether through the spread of wireless devices or generational shifts (Fox 2009)

The report describes e-patients as "high-speed and mobile," with more broadband than dial-up users (88 percent versus 72 percent) and more wireless than wired users (89 percent versus 40 percent) searching online for health information. More women than men search online for health information, as do more whites than African-Americans or Hispanics. Younger people search online more than older people do (although the percentage in the various age groups does not drop below 50 percent until the over-65 group), those with some college or a college degree search more than those without a degree, and those with higher household incomes search more than those with lower household incomes (but the percentage of use drops below 50 percent only for households with annual incomes lower than $30K, and even then, the percentage is 44 percent) (Fox 2009). The five health topics most researched online (in descending order) are:

1. a specific disease or problem

2. a specific medical treatment or procedure

3. exercise and treatment

4. doctors and other healthcare professionals

5. prescriptions and over-the-counter medications (Fox 2009)

Sixty-one percent of adults have looked online for information about one or more of the 12 health topics they were asked about (Fox 2009) Given these data, it is no surprise that at conferences and workshops, clinicians report that patients come to see them with stacks of printouts, asking such questions as, "Shouldn't we try this medication?" or "What about this approach?" For many patients, the Internet has become the de facto second opinion.

But keep in mind that much of this Internet activity is related to a person managing his health; that is, staying healthy. Just a few of the smartphone applets among the thousands now available and the many under development include fitness programs, calorie tracking, nutritional guidance, exercise training, menstrual and fertility calendars, pregnancy monitoring, mental exercises, insomnia aides, running and jogging management, hypnosis, meditation and relaxation, smoking cessation, detoxification, eye tests, triage, yoga, blood pressure tracking and analysis, blood sugar and diabetes control, how to live healthier, and how to self-assess signs and symptoms.

What does this mean for clinicians, and what impact will this have on future health information management? Clinicians must accept, and hopefully appreciate, that they are not their patients' sole resource and, instead, welcome their patients as their partners in assessing their healthcare status and treatment options. When a patient has a question to which the clinician does not have an immediate answer, the physician can guide the patient through online research to find the answer. As more and more patients arrive for their appointments with Internet-generated information, physicians must recognize the power of the Internet as the second opinion that patients routinely seek out independently. More and more physicians themselves are turning to the Internet to research symptoms and conditions.

Indeed, another aspect of mHealth is the potential that browsers offer to providers to become better informed and to provide better services. The range of guidelines, protocols, and other medical resources is substantial. In addition to Internet information resources, clinicians are increasingly accessing decision support software and other functionalities through the Internet browser. Many EMR systems are designed as ASP that allow much of the computing to be done via the Internet at the main server so that the receiving computer or mDevice is in a sense, a "dumb terminal"; that is, one without its own computer processing power but that sends and receives data to/from a host computer or "smart terminal." Not only are browsers used to access patient information, health information, and eligibility information, but also they give access to other related information. For example, a physician may view the most current, valid advance directives of a patient. Again, this is an opportunity for HIM professionals to play a major role in regard to privacy, access rights, and data integrity issues.

mDevices also enable medication management by allowing the clinician to select the appropriate medication from formularies at the point of care. Further, applets are available on mDevices such as the iPhone that show size, shape, and color of specific medications, an important enhancement when the patient doesn't know the name of a medication she is taking and brings a sample to the care setting. mDevice software applications also can identify potential adverse drug reactions. As previously noted, mDevices also can be used to remind patients of their medication schedule. This may be offered as a paid or courtesy service by the provider, or the patient may have his own mDevice application that can be set up to give medication and other reminders.

Several ePrescribing systems are offered on mDevices. The issues with small keyboards and touch screens are data integrity and authentication. It is important that such systems allow the clinician to review the prescription and authenticate it by digitally signing it before sending it off. Receiving pharmacies, in turn, must have systems that alert them to inconsistencies and potential inaccuracies, as well as to potential risks or drug interactions with other medications the patient is taking (and which the prescribing physician may not be aware of) and connect them with the prescribing physician for clarification and confirmation as needed to assure patient safety.

Table 2.2 summarizes traditional and new, Internet-based resources for clinicians.

These developments also offer new career opportunities for HIM professionals who may serve as Internet guides for patients, directing them to appropriate Web sites and preparing online bibliographies and links in their enterprise's Web site. HIM professionals also may serve as research assistants to clinicians—as Internet-age librarians. Certainly the HIM professional's correspondence role is leading to managing e-mail and text communications with patients as described earlier.

HIM professionals are in a unique position to prepare and maintain a library of resource information. They can guide patients to the most reliable Internet sources and aid them in incorporating their mDevice application-generated information into their PHR and/or EMR. For example, a new section in EMRs as well as other medical records could collect and organize patient- and device-generated

TABLE 2.2   Traditional and new resources for clinicians

Traditional Resources for Clinicians	New Resources for Clinicians
Scientific knowledge in memory	Clinician supplements and updates knowledge by instant access to the wealth of scientific information available on the Internet.
Formularies on PCs and in books. Also on some dedicated mDevices.	Clinician uses mDevice to look up formularies and related applications at the point of care and remotely.
Research in medical books and journals in office or medical library	Clinician uses mDevice to research worldwide resources.
Staff researches eligibility of services.	Clinician or staff researches eligibility at point of care prior to, upon, or during patient's office visit.
Clinician relies on his own judgment or seeks follow-up advice from specialists.	Clinician uses mDevice at point of care to consult specialists in real time while with the patient or following the visit.
Clinician has little or no information about advance directives.	Clinician uses mDevice to access information about advance directives and may be able to link to their precise wording.
Clinician calls or writes colleagues about specific diseases, treatments, or patients.	Clinician accesses worldwide experts through online professional communities.

Source: Waegemann and Tessier 2009b.

health information. The mDevice is the key enabler for this new development as low-cost, easy-to-use health software is stimulating people of all ages to seek out, record, and transmit health information over their mobile phones.

Application Cluster 3: Point-of-Care Documentation

Healthcare documentation is currently one of the most complex areas of healthcare record management, and its importance cannot be overstated. Accurate, accessible, and shareable health information is a well-accepted prerequisite to good healthcare. A wide range of documentation options exist, including handwriting, direct computer entry, dictation and transcription, natural language understanding, touch screen entry, and front-end speech recognition. Documentation is also a very expensive component of our healthcare system. Medical transcription alone, for example, requires hundreds of thousands of medical transcriptionists to meet the demand and creates an industry of over $20 billion annually. Yet the healthcare system in the United States continues to accept illegible handwriting and other documentation practices that diminish the quality of healthcare documentation by reducing accuracy, accessibility, and shareability. Indeed, the documentation hurdles encountered with EMR systems are major factors accounting for their slow implementation.

mHealth devices offer opportunities for improving documentation, but they will require major changes in skills and practices as clinicians learn how to use the mDevice. The clinician must make the entry, review the entry, edit as needed, and sign off accordingly, all within seconds and without outside intervention. HIM professionals are finding that many clinicians are already embracing the potential of mDevices as documentation tools, others are more cautious and slow to move toward adoption, and still others are resistant. Some older physicians may reject the idea of using an mDevice for documentation due to the small screen, the small keyboard, and the needed adjustment in work style and workflow. In such cases, tablets may be more attractive. The advantages and disadvantages of light weight and small screen versus heavier weight and large screen need to be explained and experimented with. Ultimately, the choice of whether or not to use such devices will, for the most part, fall to the individual user. But it is anticipated that even some reluctant and resistant individuals may be wooed to this revolutionary device when they see the benefits it offers both providers and patients.

In discussing healthcare documentation, it is important to address its two parts: information capture and report generation. Information capture is the process of recording representations of human thought, perceptions, or actions in documenting patient care, as well as device-generated information that is gathered and/or computed about a patient as part of healthcare. Typical means for information capture are handwriting, speaking, typing, touching a screen, or pointing and clicking on words or phrases. Other means include videotaping, audio recording, and image generation through x-rays. While the main tools of information capture on wireless mobile devices are a keyboard, a screen, and perhaps a stylus (but for the increasingly common touch screen, a finger), speech recognition is being used more frequently as well. Report generation follows information capture and includes the construction of a healthcare document through formatting and/or structuring the captured information. It includes analyzing, organizing, and presenting captured patient information for authentication and inclusion in the patient's healthcare record. Digital report generation is the software approach that organizes and displays the captured information as desired or required.

There is no question that information capture through mDevices is affecting health information management professionals in their core activities. The digital capture of structured text is already moving some clinicians away from free text documentation. Of course, chart assembly, storage, retrieval, and related activities take on a whole new meaning in the digital healthcare record world. Further, digital signatures added at the end of the documentation process are replacing wet signatures, and traditional transcription is very slowly being replaced by real-time documentation in those sections of reports that allow structured entry (for example, diagnoses, medications, lab data) and very likely by speech recognition (front-end or back-end) in those sections that are more dependent on free text (for example, history of present illness).

Direct mDevice input by keyboard or touch-screen keyboard, stylus, projected keyboard, scanned images, scanned bar codes and other repeatable codes, speech recognition, photos, or clinical imaging, as well as their hybrids, must be managed to assure it meets the essential requirements of health documentation.

Many steps must be taken to create systems and policies that make healthcare documentation more efficient and effective for quality healthcare as clinicians increasingly use mDevices. The essential principles of healthcare documentation as defined by the Consensus Workgroup on Health Information Capture and Report Generation (2002) require unique patient identification within and across healthcare documentation systems. In addition, the healthcare documentation must be accurate and consistent, complete, timely, interoperable across types of documentation systems, accessible at any time and at any place where patient care is needed, auditable, and confidential and secure, with appropriate authentication and accountability.

The practitioner who effectively interacts with electronic resources for patient care, rather than relying on memory, gains more complete and timely access to information. Rapid access to databases such as formularies, drug references, and other decision-making support tools, improves the quality of care. When this is accompanied by practices that support the essential principles of healthcare documentation noted above, quality of care is further enhanced.

In summary, mHealth is causing a revolution in healthcare. It is changing communication, transforming work patterns and affecting clinicians, patients, and many others. For health information management, the most important feature of healthcare documentation with mDevices is that it occurs at the point of care. This use of mDevices for documentation in the exam room or at the bedside of a patient adds a whole new dimension to health information management.

Table 2.3 summarizes how traditional healthcare documentation is changing and its impact on HIM.

Application Cluster 4: Disease Management

The most promising part of the mHealth Revolution is communication-based disease management. It is at the heart of the disruptive nature of communication-based care patterns. The combination of participatory health and mHealth as its enabling technology promises to deliver better care at a reduced cost. Although few controlled studies have been published, the results of a number of proprietary studies have shown that the use of this technology results in better care and decreased costs. In one published study, patients who were actively involved in their care through cell phone communications had a 2.03 percentage-point drop in their glycated hemoglobin (Hb1Ac) level (Quinn et al. 2008).

Among mHealth application clusters, disease management has the strongest potential to change behavior and improve health. Patient data, such as daily glucometer readings for diabetic patients, are sent directly to the provider to offer continuous rather than periodic monitoring and thus more timely intervention. Some applications offer patients the opportunity to maintain food and exercise diaries as well as self-observations. They also provide prompts when lifestyle changes, such as diet adjustments, result in improved readings. Other conditions where such applications have produced astounding results include asthma, dermatology,

TABLE 2.3 How healthcare documentation is changing and its impact on HIM

Traditional Documentation	New Documentation Patterns	Impact on HIM
Handwriting and dictation for transcription.	Direct mDevice documentation by voice (speech recognition or transcription), keyboard, or touch screen entry by clinician	Principles of documentation must be enforced in new systems, with special attention to hybrid systems.
Limited documentation options in the exam room.	Clinician uses mDevice in exam room, hospital ward, at bedside, or anywhere to document in real time at point of care or remotely.	Systems for synchronization and data integrity must be designed and implemented. Confidentiality and security of PHI must be assured.
Little standardization. Free text. Proliferation of customized templates.	Increasingly standardized, structured text entry, integrated with free text where required.	Documentation standards must be monitored. Clinicians must be educated and guided.
Documentation completed after the visit (sometimes long after).	Documentation completed at time of visit through real-time data entry	Documentation standards must be monitored and integrated into patient records.
Text is routinely edited by medical transcriptionists or other medical editors.	Documentation is not regularly reviewed by others.	Systems must be monitored. Random audits must be scheduled.
Signature is added after transcription.	Digital signature in real time as documentation is completed.	Implementation of authentication and data integrity must be assured.

Source: Waegemann and Tessier 2009c.

preventive care in pregnancy, smoking cessation, and hypertension. Numerous other disease management programs are under development.

Consider a patient with hypertension. If he sees his physician every few weeks to check his blood pressure, each reading potentially will be affected by the "white coat syndrome," meaning a patient's blood pressure commonly increases when the reading is done by a doctor or nurse. Further, if he had to wait a long time in the waiting room and is anxious about missing his professional appointments, his blood pressure is likely to be abnormally high. Now consider the alternative. A patient routinely takes his blood pressure at home in an everyday environment and records it via Bluetooth directly into his PHR through his cell phone. These data are much more reliable, and they can show trends over time that relate to the patient's everyday life and not just to sporadic readings in the physician's office.

Communication-based disease management increases the quality of care, decreases costs, provides better insights for clinicians, and gives patients a feeling of being cared for between visits to the provider's office. The cell phone and other electronic devices enable a completely different communication pattern between patients and clinicians. Of course, such communication is not limited to mDevices but may be conducted via regular (landline) phones, home monitors, TV sets, or other telemedicine devices and systems as well. In other words, this new communication pattern takes a good part of patient care out of the clinician's office and puts it into the home or, when facilitated by mDevices, to wherever the patient is—in a bus or car, visiting relatives, shopping, on vacation, or anywhere.

While this new communication pattern of healthcare will develop gradually and may not be fully implemented across provider settings for a few years, the trend is clear and is not likely to be reversed.

mDevice-enabled disease management creates the potential for communication between patients and clinicians that is not limited to specific visits or services. Rather, it may occur 24/7—at any time of the day or night on work days and weekends. This creates a new challenge for health information management as systems must be designed that screen incoming information according to medical urgency and sort such messages into those that:

- Can be handled by canned, standard responses

- Require timely and customized, but nonurgent responses from a nurse practitioner or other healthcare professional, much like telephone inquiries are currently handled

- Allow time-flexible responses that a provider or his representative can give at his own convenience, for instance, in the evening or when workflow allows

- Require immediate attention; that is, those that are urgent or emergencies

To further complicate matters, the communication may come not from the patient himself but from someone else involved in the patient's care. In the past, it was unthinkable that a mother would show up for her child's pediatric visit without the child. Now the mother may communicate by e-mail with health professionals without the child's direct involvement. In other instances, a relative, a neighbor, a friend, or other person may seek help for a person, with authorization, of course.

Perhaps even more revolutionary, is the possibility that the child himself will directly contact the provider, especially as the child enters adolescence and as younger children have greater access to cell phones. Children may engage in such communications with or without their parents' knowledge. It will be important for pediatricians and other providers to work with both the children and their parents to assure which direct communications between provider and child are appropriate and authorized. In the case of a child with diabetes or asthma, for example, their disease management very likely will deliberately involve direct communications between the child and the provider.

mDevice-based disease management communication also facilitates access to guidelines and protocols at the point of care. Many applets are available on smartphones such as the iPhone, Blackberry, and G1 Android that offer guidance in the care process, help with management issues such as formularies, enable orders, and many other functions.

On the patients' side, many mDevices that monitor and capture information will allow them to record vital signs and other body-generated information that help them to better manage their disease. Several disease management programs are already available for such conditions as diabetes, asthma, hypertension, smoking cessation, dermatology, and obstetrics. More are anticipated in the near future, as are developments to make such devices even more functional. For instance, at present, diabetes patients are using glucose monitoring devices and insulin delivery pumps. In the future, such devices will be able to capture information and send it to the provider's EMR as well as to the patient's PHR. In addition, such devices will provide communication options, behavioral guidelines, nutritional information, and other functionalities. Some will even autoinject insulin when the patient's blood sugar drops below a certain point. Additional mApplications are available that provide patients with daily allergy alerts, such as pollen counts. Others can scan grocery products to identify ingredients and alert the patient to the particular ingredients to which they are allergic.

It is obvious that this is the beginning of a new era of healthcare and disease management. This means HIM management must prepare for and adjust to the new challenges that such developments present.

Application Cluster 5: Education Programs and Telemedicine

The new world of education and on-the-job training via cell phones is opening up many applications in various healthcare professions. Medical schools are increasingly using mDevices in their educational programs, with downloaded applications replacing texts and real-time access to resources such as formularies and disease management guidelines. Medical schools also offer student evaluations and reviews of instructors and texts. Nursing education and on-the-job training are additional areas in which mDevices are being used successfully.

mDevices allow participants in widely scattered locations to share educational activities, share data, and view live or recorded videos simultaneously over the Internet without being together in a classroom or at a PC. This opens up undreamed of opportunities both for scheduled, structured educational programs and for ad hoc, spontaneous, real-time, point-of-care educational opportunities for clinicians as well as patients.

mDevices in developing countries offer telemedicine observations and treatments that are not available otherwise. Some of these countries don't have the infrastructure for EMRs. Indeed, in some instances, they don't even have paper medical records. So mDevice communication allows them to leapfrog the bureaucracy, requirements, and shortcomings of EMRs and to provide education and treatment simply and directly, because mDevices, unlike EMRs, are widely interoperable and can easily, readily, and quickly connect and exchange data.

In the United States, it is anticipated that mDevices will allow indigent populations and others without the means for routine care to at least communicate for emergency and urgent care and, at best, to access wellness and treatment programs designed specifically to reach such populations. Even those with full health insurance and generally easy access to healthcare could find themselves in circumstances where telemedicine through mDevices could guide immediate treatment until more traditional care is available.

George Washington Medical Faculty Associates has developed what it calls the "Back-up Brain" education series for clinical professionals, defining the back-up brain as any device that helps clinicians in their daily routine, allowing them to reference complex data points and enabling them to "think, process, and clear" with "stream of consciousness thinking" through notes and reminders that pop up, are recorded, and then cleared to make way for the next "think, process, and clear" round (Stern 2009).

Application Cluster 6: Professional Communication

New communication methods also allow clinicians and their peers and colleagues to more easily discuss, for example, rare cases or the outcome of specific patient populations, such as the progress of diabetes patients. Such provider-based information communities could create a new role for local, regional, and national professional and specialty societies. With more social networking on the Internet, including through mDevices, HIM professionals must prepare for professional networking that is already beginning to be adopted and is expected to grow tremendously in the not-too-distant future.

Within hospitals and other care organizations, mobile phone systems are already enabling nurses to reduce waste, implement on-the-job training, and be more efficient in their daily tasks as shown in some current projects (McLeod 2009). The implementation of these workflow changes requires that professional education must take place and guidelines must be established. Much of such mDevice use involves patient care documentation, and the HIM professional can work with the nursing department to promote its adoption, both for efficiency and to improve patient care and assure integration.

mDevices also can be used to facilitate team conferences about a patient's status and treatment if all team members are not required or able to be physically present. mDevice-based calls offering voice, data, and video transmission allow anyone to participate, anytime, anywhere. This can be particularly important in situations where key specialists may not be able to reach the bedside in time to contribute their expertise.

Application Cluster 7: Administrative Applications

Asset Tracking

As noted earlier, some mApplications can scan barcodes. Still others are based on radio frequency identification (RFID) systems, which unlike barcode scanning, do not require line-of-sight reading and can be done at greater distances. In provider institutions, these scanning processes facilitate management of medical and surgical supplies and equipment, reducing incidents of loss and theft as well as time lost in searching for them.

Enhancing Security through mDevice-Tracking mDevices

There are tracking applications for the mDevices themselves, so when they are lost or stolen, their location can be determined. These applications also allow the mDevices to be wiped clean, deleting identification and content, and deactivating security codes. They also facilitate confirmation that all devices in the inventory are present and accounted for. These are all important applications for the health information manager to be aware of and to require in order to protect patient privacy and confidentiality.

Patient Flow Management

mDevices with RFID or bar coding capabilities also can enhance patient flow management, providing more complete and real-time data for activities like admissions/discharges, bed assignments, and scheduling. Where medical records are still primarily accessed in paper form, tracking patient records in these ways can be a real benefit and can contribute to patient flow management by assuring the patient's record and its relevant contents are accessible when and where the patient is seen, diminishing the delay factor resulting from hunts for misfiled charts and their contents.

Patient Identification

In 1998, in response to strong opposition among privacy experts against efforts to adopt a national patient identifier, the U.S. Congress passed legislation prohibiting such a patient identification system, and it does not appear likely that they will soon reverse that position. So provider institutions remain responsible for both developing their own patient ID systems and finding means to accurately and consistently uniquely identify a patient, to assure multiple identifications of a single patient are merged accurately, to assure a patient's information from multiple sources with multiple identifications is accurately merged, and to protect against medical identify theft. The adoption of EMRs, which are expected to support these efforts, frequently falls short.

The same requirements for patient identification in paper records and electronic records apply to mHealth records and communications, and again HIM professionals will be tasked with assuring that these requirements and the obligations to patient privacy and confidentiality are met. With the advent of PHRs, patient awareness of these concerns and expectations will increase, and HIM professionals in particular are likely to encounter circumstances where a patient will authorize access to some parts of his paper record, EMR, or PHR to some providers (and others, such as family members) at the same time that he restricts access to all or parts of these same records to other individuals.

A few years ago, an important effort to assist in patient identification began within ASTM International (the nation's oldest standards development organization) when its E31 Committee on Health Informatics developed a standard for a voluntary universal health identifier (VUHID). The standard describes the necessary principles to design a VUHID system "to enable unambiguous identification of individuals in order to facilitate the delivery of healthcare" (ASTM 2007). This VUHID standard is complementary to another ASTM standard, E1714-07 Standard Guide for Properties of a Universal Healthcare Identifier (UHID) (ASTM 2007).

Since then, a not-for-profit organization, Global Patient Identifiers, Inc. (GPII) has been formed as a sponsor of VUHID, with the goal of making "unique healthcare identifiers available to any patient who uses the services of a regional health information organization (RHIO) or health information exchange (HIE) to:

- Enable error-free linkages of clinical information across provider sites;

- Enhance patient control over the privacy of their information;

- Improve the quality of medical care and the efficiency of its delivery;

- Reduce medical errors related to mis-identification of patients;

- Decrease incidents of healthcare-related identity theft; and

- Help control healthcare costs as a result of these impacts" (GPII2009).

GPII is establishing business relationships to offer and administer VUHID programs nationally and potentially internationally. It offers two types of voluntary identifiers: the open voluntary identifier (OVID) that links a patient's demographic records across systems and the private (anonymous) voluntary identifier (PVID) that can tag sensitive medical information to control who has access to that information and who can identify the patient associated with that information (GPII 2009).

The key features of the VUHID, of course, are that it is:

- Voluntary, so there is no requirement for anyone to use it, thus staying within the boundaries of Congressional action.

- Secure, offering compliance with privacy and confidentiality concerns and requirements of both patients and providers.

The VUHID's major shortcoming is the complexity of its secure identification codes.

While VUHID is not required for mHealth PHR or other patient applications on mDevices, it holds great potential for enabling patients to more easily connect and communicate with multiple clinicians and provider sites. Therefore, it should be given serious attention by HIM professionals. Indeed some may find this a unique opportunity to take the lead in offering VUHID to patients served by their institution.

Communication with Patient's Support Parties

mDevices can facilitate provider communications with patient's support parties, including family members, clergy, and healthcare proxies. Of course, such communications must be authorized by the patient, so here again is an opportunity for HIM professionals to work with an institution to offer nonclinical but important programs to patients who often are concerned about how their family and others can be contacted and informed, according to their own preferences.

Application Cluster 8: Financial Applications

mDevices can connect patients and payers as well as payers and providers. Before a patient receives care, their eligibility and coverage can be communicated directly to them and their providers, and where real-time charge capture is being implemented, the payer can notify both the patient and provider of the total covered by insurance as well as the copayment required of the patient. Additionally, payers can send notices directly to subscribers' cell phones of payments due or past due, as well as changes in their policies. Applications are also available for checking ICD and other codes in the exam room, for example, and forwarding them to the billing office. This not only streamlines the billing process but also improves it as the applications may prompt or remind the clinician to be more specific in coding, for example, noting complications with diabetes that she might otherwise have neglected to address either in the assessment or in the coding.

Payment by cell phone is also likely to become a part of patients' (and their healthcare providers') daily financial transactions. "The aim is to turn (cell) phones into virtual credit cards or checkbooks, enabling the kind of click-and-buy commerce and online banking that people have come to expect on their PCs" (Miller and Richtel 2009). Such mDevice-based transactions are already implemented in some European countries, where public transportation, for example, can be paid for by one's cell phone. Even some current mDevices in the United States facilitate payments for purchases (such as music downloads) because the mDevice applications are linked to pre-existing online user accounts, including those specific to a business (for example, Apple), those linked to credit cards, and those linked to banking accounts.

Application Cluster 9: Emergency Care

Emergency medical services (EMS) traditionally include collecting data on the patient while en route to the emergency center and delivering it in a completed paper form upon arrival. The mDevice can significantly enhance this process. In cities such as San Diego, EMS providers are using mDevices to collect patient information and send it wirelessly in advance to the emergency center, facilitating faster and more informed triaging. Their system has reportedly saved $2.5 million per annum and many lives (Pringle 2008). In the future, such systems may access information that is stored on the patient's cell phone, such as the PHR, or directly identify and contact the patient's primary care provider to both inform him and get more information about the patient. Thus, mHealth enables the patient's relevant history and current status to be more readily available to the emergency center for assessment and decision-making. HIM professionals must ensure that patient information communicated through mDevices to the Emergency Department is incorporated into the patient's medical record.

Application Cluster 10: Public Health

mHealth enables the integration of personal health and public health. mDevices allow disease reporting, surveillance, and notification of the patient population in emergency situations such as pandemics or threat of bioterrorism or disasters, whether natural or man-made.

Disease reporting surveillance reveals how many people in a given region show the same symptoms and how they respond to treatment. Such disease reporting with cell phones is already being used successfully in a number of regions, particularly in Africa.

Additionally, in the case of disasters, whether natural or man-made, mDevices can quickly and easily contact and connect responsible personnel, both within the physical facility and scattered throughout the city, state, country, or globe, enabling them both to be informed and to collaborate on handling the crisis.

If a specific population were threatened with an infectious disease or bioterrorism, the goals would be to notify thousands of clinicians or citizens about the threat, to give guidance on appropriate behavior, and/or encourage victims to visit healthcare facilities, including public health stations. Similarly, the data would provide clinicians and public health officials with guidance on the degree of the threat and its trends, better enabling them to respond appropriately.

Public health applications on mDevices increasingly are being integrated into the care process. At present, their use is greater in underdeveloped countries, but it is expected that adoption will become pervasive worldwide as the value and simplicity of mDevice-based, real-time disease surveillance and disaster response, for example, are contrasted with the slower, more traditional systems, some of which remain paper-based and manual in terms of both reporting and interpreting.

Application 11: Pharma/Clinical Trials

The use of cell phones in clinical trials is not new. At least since 2003, pharmaceutical companies have been giving patients cell phones to use for reporting during clinical trials. These mDevice-based systems have become more sophisticated and are not limited to small population groups, and when the data are automatically collected through built-in systems, they are considered more reliable than manually entered data which may, deliberately or not, be skewed by the patient.

Further, as disease-specific patient groups exchange their experiences with specific medications or treatment plans, data are being collected from patients who might otherwise not have been reached in the past, creating what some refer to as ad hoc clinical trials. While there is legitimate concern that such ad hoc groups are not designed properly as clinical trials (that is, they do not include control groups and double-blind trials), the value of their input is nevertheless being recognized. Certainly such voluntary information exchange, with patients comparing their experiences and alerting each other to interactions or failed treatment attempts, will not replace sophisticated, rigidly designed trials, but also they are not likely to be suppressed.

Application Cluster 12: Body Area Networks (BAN)

Body area networks involve implanted or wearable computer devices that communicate or exchange data with nearby IT devices. They can be particularly beneficial in healthcare when they monitor such things as heart rate and rhythm in order to alert the patient and provider to an impending heart attack, or when they monitor a patient's blood sugar and autoinject insulin when it drops to a predefined value. This may at first glance seem futuristic, but already devices worn by patients are transmitting vital signs on an ongoing basis, and band aids with tiny communication clips are giving clinicians clues to the healing process. Today's applications are the tip of the iceberg for this rapidly developing field, which will require HIM professionals to ensure that such information is appropriately entered into the patient's record.

Impact on Healthcare and HIMs

As extensive as this review of the application clusters is, it barely touches on the more than 5,000 mDevice health-related applications available today. The number and variety of applications within each cluster are growing, and perhaps additional clusters will be identified. This means that healthcare as we have known it for so long—as patients, as clinicians, as HIM professionals, and as payers and others—is changing in many ways that were and will continue to be unanticipated. It is inevitable, then, that all these stakeholders in healthcare will be affected by it. The HIM professional's response to it will determine not so much the success of mHealth but the success and growth of the profession itself.

CHAPTER 3

Patients' and Consumers' Personal Health Records: mDevices and Applications

Introduction

No one argues against the fact that a comprehensive patient record would improve the quality of care immensely by giving each practitioner a complete overview of a person's healthcare status and treatment. Yet, after decades of effort, that goal remains elusive. This is one of the reasons why millions of people are collecting copies of their healthcare records from providers and feeding them into their Web-based personal health record (PHR). Many people do this not only for themselves but also for their children and their elderly relatives and others for whom they are responsible.

The concept of personal health records is decades old. It is driven by two goals. The first goal is to get patients more involved in and educated about their healthcare status and treatment based on the belief that, with their own copy of their health records, patients can better understand, participate in, and manage their healthcare, and they can share their health records as needed and at their discretion. The second goal has developed more recently, as the quest for electronic medical records (EMRs) flounders and there is increasing patient awareness and concern that physicians and other practitioners often provide patient care without knowing what has been done previously by whom. This leads to wasteful duplication and to clinical decision-making that does not take into account critical data related to patient health because it is not available in real time at the point of care. With interoperability among EMR systems, and therefore among providers, not yet a reality, patients themselves can take the critical role of providing their relevant information to clinicians from one provider site to another and from one encounter to another. Imagine a patient whose health information is stored at 18 different provider locations, few or none of them connected or interoperable and none assuring timely communication about a patient's status. Patients cannot understand why their primary care facility and other provider sites where they are seen require them to repeatedly provide the same demographic and insurance information, why the results of laboratory work done following one visit are not readily available to the consulting physician for assessment and decision-making, potentially necessitating additional costly visits. No wonder that patients are increasingly motivated to take their health information into their own hands in order to create one place where relevant aspects of their health information can be readily and easily accessed.

The first personal health record systems came to market in the 1970s. Simple software programs facilitated patients' entering their health data. Soon it became apparent that such PHRs should be portable so that patients could take the information to their providers. Initially, such information was stored on smart cards, particularly in the military and in Europe, but smart cards need an infrastructure of special card readers and other equipment that can be costly to purchase and frustrating to use, particularly if the intended recipient does not have compatible equipment. In the late 1990s, compact disks (CDs) became a popular medium. With the acceptance of the USB drive as a universal portable storage device, hopes arose that this would be the ideal medium for PHRs, since it was easily portable and compatible with any computer with a USB port.

In 2004, at the national conference Towards the Electronic Patient Record (TEPR), approximately 2,000 USB drives with a mock data set (the Continuity of Care Record or CCR) were distributed to conference attendees to demonstrate the value of the data set itself as well as its portability. Subsequently, however, as reported at the TEPR 2007 conference, patients who had their PHR information on a USB drive were unsuccessful in sharing the stored information with clinics and hospitals because emergency rooms and practices were not willing to take the risk of inserting such a device into their computers for fear of contracting viruses. Although USB drives that allow encryption and have better security are now available, they remain suspect. So a nonintrusive mDevice might be more readily accepted.

There are many versions of PHRs. Many providers now have patient portals that allow the patient to see some of their health information. These passive portals might focus on medication lists and allergies or on appointments and care plans, but they do not allow the patient to actively record information, and so their status as PHRs is disputed. We are moving toward a more complex PHR, one that is controlled by the patient but that also includes authenticated medical information documented by a healthcare provider with protection against its alteration. In addition to a few dozen very small PHR companies, a number of major providers offer their own versions of PHRs, with the Veterans Administration and Kaiser Permanente among those with the most users. Microsoft HealthVault and Google Health also have made major inroads. Google is a more open system that allows greater patient input, while Microsoft HealthVault is focused on creating an ecosystem that allows some interoperability with providers and facilitates synchronization of various versions. Microsoft is moving toward integrating the mobile phone into its ecosystem, while Project HealthDesign reports, "Among the most common PHR platforms, only Google Health has a meaningful iPhone presence" (Rothstein and Ricciardi, 2009).

For some years, the telecommunications industry has been moving toward launching the cell phone as a major healthcare tool, not only to carry patient health histories but also to bring a variety of functions to the caregiver, patient, payer, and even to pharmaceutical companies. At the TEPR 2008 conference, one company demonstrated a system that allows any patient to download his relevant insurance and health data onto almost any cell phone and safely and securely transmit it when needed. Other companies offer or are developing similar systems, and there is increasing interest in cell phone–based PHR implementations, which will enable patient-controlled, easy, and secure access, entry, and transmission of healthcare information anywhere, anytime (Waegemann 2009c).

Consensus on the Data Set

The original hopes for quick implementation of such PHRs on the cell phone quickly evaporated due to several hurdles that must be overcome before the PHR on the phone application will get widespread adoption. The first is an agreement on a universal data set. The answer for many PHR deliverers, from major industry leaders such as Microsoft and Google, to small, independent companies and just about everything in between (for example, payers, doctors offices, hospitals, and employers) has been ASTM International's Continuity of Care (CCR) industry standard specification (ASTM 2005), a comprehensive data set of the most relevant current and past information about a patient's healthcare status and treatment. The data set includes 17 categories of information that should, if relevant, be included for a particular patient. Even when the PHR is not based on the CCR, these same categories of patient information should be included in some form or another if the PHR is to adequately meet the patient's needs and those of healthcare providers with whom they may share their PHR. In summary form, these 17 categories are:

- **Payers**—Eligibility, coverage, contact information, etc.
- **Advance directive**s—Do they exist? If so, what are they and where can they be accessed?
- **Nonhealthcare support**—family, clergy, legal representative, etc
- **Functional status**—Activities of daily living, ambulatory status, etc.
- **Problems**—Symptoms, diagnoses, conditions, etc.
- **Family history**—Genetic or familial information relevant to the patient's health status
- **Social history**—Marital status, employment, drug/alcohol use, etc.
- **Alerts**—Allergies, drug interactions, other types of alerts, etc.
- **Medications**—Prescription and over-the-counter drugs, herbals, vitamins, etc., including details of dosage, route, and form as well as fulfillment history

- **Medical equipment**—Internal and external medical devices
- **Immunizations**—When, what, reactions, etc.
- **Vital signs**—The usual, plus any findings relevant to the patient or specialty (for example, head circumference for newborns)
- **Results**—Lab, x-ray, etc.
- **Therapeutic and diagnostic procedures**
- **History-based encounters**
- **Future plan of care**
- **Healthcare providers**—Names and contact information for all relevant healthcare providers

The CCR is unique both because of its simplicity and because it was developed primarily by physicians for physicians; that is, experts in clinical care and content determined what constitutes the essential patient data set. Under the leadership of ASTM E31 Committee on Healthcare Informatics, the CCR task group's work was co-sponsored by leading medical/specialty societies, including the American Medical Association, the American Academy of Family Physicians, the American Academy of Pediatrics, the Massachusetts Medical Society (a past president of which co-chairs the ASTM CCR task group, along with the author of this text), and several other professional and industry organizations. These participants asked themselves this question: If I or another clinician were to see this patient for the first time, what information about her healthcare status and treatment is essential to know in order to assure continuity of care? Initially, the developers anticipated the primary use for the CCR would be for referrals and discharges, but it quickly became obvious that its utility extends far beyond that to school health, eldercare, initial population of EMRs (in place of, or supplemented by, selective scanning), disaster planning (think Katrina), and, of course, PHRs.

Currently, the majority of PHR systems are based on the CCR with its W3C XML schema because this state-of-the-art technology facilitates interoperability. Additionally, the CCR data set is available as a continuity of care document (CCD) for HL7 messaging-based systems, thus enabling such EMR systems to offer it as well.

Consensus on the Communication System

Developing and agreeing on an industry standard data set is one thing. Implementing the data set on the cell phone is another matter entirely. Any patient is entitled to ask for a copy of her medical record, but how does she get it onto her cell phone? Assume a patient receives a stack of paper with a combination of printed and handwritten information. How can such information be organized, authenticated, and displayed in a user-friendly format so that it makes sense, particularly on the phone? A patient's challenge is to gather the information from copies of his medical records from a variety of sources and to create a concise CCR data set from it. This is an overwhelming task for most patients, and it is also fraught with authenticity problems. A major obstacle is that some physicians do not trust a data set that has been developed and maintained by the patient, despite their lifelong experience of accepting patients' descriptions of symptoms and history when they meet with them in their practice. In any case, it is essential that the PHR data set include, in addition to data originated or recorded by the patient himself, authenticated data that is originated by caregivers, and that such data remain in authenticated, "read only" format so that the patient cannot change it.

This means that the "official" data should come from a provider or other authority. Some companies have taken the approach that the first data set should come from the payer and should be based on services that were paid for. However, many physicians and patients oppose this approach, saying that payer information cannot be trusted for either completeness or accuracy and that it gives a partial picture at best and a distorted one at worst. Proponents of this approach respond to such criticism by pointing out that it is better to get authenticated payer information than to have nothing, and the provider can correct/amend incorrect or incomplete information when the patient presents her PHR for the first time. This topic encountered another twist recently when it was reported that a patient found out that his billing codes, instead of doctors' diagnoses, were transmitted to Google Health and, as a result, his Google Health PHR portrayed his status incorrectly (Kolakowski 2009).

Ideally, the PHR's basic CCR data set should come from the healthcare provider. Neither the patient nor anyone else should be allowed to edit or alter such information except with appropriate authority and through appropriate procedures for amending patient care documentation. Information provided directly by the patient must be labeled as such. Indeed, one of the important features of a fully implemented CCR is that the source of each data element can be identified.

There also must be a consensus on the communication system. First, any cell phone should be able to accommodate and communicate the data set. Also, any telecommunications carrier (such as AT&T, Verizon, Sprint, T-Mobile) must be able to transmit the data securely. To sum up, the communication system should be device-neutral and carrier-neutral, thus supporting interoperability across devices and carriers.

It is important to coordinate the systems that integrate the PHR/CCR with the EMR system or other health IT (HIT) systems. This means that any clinic, hospital, nursing home, or doctor's office must be able to import or export the data set, with authorization of course. If the provider does not have an EMR, the PHR information can be sent to the office as a fax. But how can an office update the information and send a copy back to the patient's phone? One solution is to have a Web-based PHR, which allows easy access and exchange between mDevices, provides links to EMRs, and houses the data in proprietary systems maintained by providers, payers, the patients themselves, or in such systems as Microsoft HealthVault and Google Health.

Why would patients want their health data held on, accessible through, or exchanged via their cell phones? Even if early versions carry only insurance data combined with patient demographic data, this has great appeal to some. Patients are tired of having to provide their information over and over again throughout the care process. Sending such information by cell phone to the provider before leaving home means the patient can expect to spend less time checking in on arrival; she will only need to confirm the institution's receipt of the information. In hospitals with silo-type departmental systems, sending information by cell phone means the patient will not have to give the information to someone in the outpatient department and then give the same information again in radiology, lab, and other departments. If allergies, medication history, and other important CCR data are documented in the data set, even better!

A newly recognized value of PHRs has been reported by Robert Wood Johnson Project HealthDesign, which notes that observations of daily living (ODL) "may be the most important feature of PHRs. ODLs are information that is collected and reported by the patient (sleep, diet, exercise, mood, adherence to medications)—information important to health, but not collected in a clinical encounter" (Brennan 2009). The point is that health cannot be managed only at clinical encounters; it must be managed on a daily basis. Further, a patient's health status cannot be assessed adequately in a single encounter or even in a series of encounters; rather, it is an ongoing phenomenon. ODLs enable patients to present a more complete picture of their health, to identify what treatments are working when, and to have more meaningful encounters with their providers when they do meet with them. At present, most health-related applications "focus overwhelmingly on collecting, tracking, analyzing, and even sharing both traditional clinical measures of health and Observations of Daily Living," but unfortunately, their integration with full PHRs lags behind and remains to be developed to its fullest potential (Rothstein and Ricciardi, 2009).

Overcoming Confidentiality, Security, and Data Protection Concerns

A PHR system can only succeed if patients trust it. When people are concerned that confidentiality may be compromised, they will not want a PHR. Thus, systems must use encryption, anyone accessing any data must be identified, the host system must be safe and secure, and adequate policies must guide the overall system. The first concern is where such data resides. Should it reside with the primary healthcare provider, an independent company, a PHR provider such as Microsoft Vault or Google Health, or the patient himself? It is likely that patients will have different preferences based on their personal attitude toward confidentiality and security, their sophistication in managing their health, their degree of participation in their healthcare, the diversity of their providers, and their trust in a PHR provider system. For HIM professionals, this means that patients should be alerted to the risks and threats, as well as the design and benefits, of the various systems, and they should be advised that the decision to have a PHR, and which type of PHR to have, is the patient's right. Of course, when the provider organization itself is involved in a PHR program, it must assure the implementation of strong security measures.

Overcoming Authentication Concerns

Physicians have stated for many years that they will only consider PHR information if it is authenticated by another physician. They do not accept any PHR information that has been tampered with by the patient. The argument that a patient may manipulate information when describing symptoms to the clinician has been repeatedly countered by the rationale that clinicians routinely use their own judgment as to which of the patient's oral statements they accept, which they question, and which they ignore or reject. Therefore, a PHR on the phone, or any PHR for that matter, should have a section where patients can enter data and comments, as well as a safeguarded section where authenticated caregiver information is displayed. Where the full extent of the CCR is used, a caregiver can identify the source of each data element and access information on how to contact that source. This kind of professional access and communication will be facilitated by and become more common in an mHealth environment.

Conclusion

PHRs are being widely developed, implemented, and adopted, as are mDevice-based health-related applications. The integration of these applications into PHRs through mDevices facilitates their access and communication, in turn stimulating participatory health throughout all strata of healthcare. The combination of all these factors is in its early stages and so is just beginning to impact the management of health records. This impact will grow and demand integration of traditional records (both paper and electronic) with mDevice-based PHRs and their related applications, including ODLs.

CHAPTER 4

Implementing mDevices in Healthcare

Introduction

The adoption of mDevices in healthcare and the consequent stimulus to participatory health pose a major challenge to HIM professionals. Development of policies and guidelines for mDevice management, as well as a long-term strategy toward participatory health, is required of any doctor's office, clinic, hospital, or other healthcare delivery system. We will briefly address developing the long-term strategy and then give greater attention to policies and guidelines.

Organizational Strategies

Developing a long-term strategy toward participatory health involves four steps:

1. Alert top management of the organization to the importance of the new developments of mHealth and participatory health, the need for new systems that allow continuous communication between patients and clinicians, and what needs to be done to create such systems, as well as how both administrative and clinical workflow will be affected.

2. Educate all stakeholders about these new system requirements and their impact on workflow, both administrative and clinical, and discuss with all stakeholders their evolving roles in the competitive healthcare market of the future.

3. Identify the extent and type of current uses of mDevices in the organization, including identification of any "no cell phone" areas, and determine the potential for extending open areas for cell phone use by clinicians, staff, patients, and visitors.

4. Develop a step-by-step implementation plan that will facilitate participatory health and new communication systems, while assuring compliance with federal and state laws and regulations, and institutional policies and procedures regarding protected health information (PHI).

Designing a WLAN Architecture for Healthcare Institutions

Designing a wireless local area network infrastructure requires five steps (Air Magnet 2009):

1. The system must be designed with healthcare applications in mind. This requires a clinical grade, robust system that can accommodate, adjust, and grow according to the facility's needs. Attention must be given to the various applications an organization currently uses and those it anticipates using. All aspects of the environment must be assessed, both in the planning stage and at least twice yearly.

2. The system must maintain "always on" reliability and performance. This requires 24/7 monitoring and both anticipating and addressing potential problems before they occur.

3. The system must protect against security threats. This requires a proactive design that protects not just patient records but also institutional records and assets. Approved and unapproved devices must be identified and controlled.

4. Compliance reporting should be automated for both the Health Insurance Portability and Accountability Act (HIPAA) and payment card industry reports for auditing purposes. The organization should keep strict records and forensic analysis of any significant event

5. For maximum efficiency, the organization must evaluate and compare in-house vs. contracted services for WLAN management, in terms of efficiency and cost.

The technical components and implementation of these requirements will come under the aegis of the IT department, but the HIM department should be informed and should contribute expertise regarding expectations and requirements related to the protection of patient information and the provision of improved communication services to all stakeholders.

Healthcare providers report increasing frustration with telecommunications carriers (such as AT&T, Verizon, T-Mobile, and Sprint) when trying to integrate all of them into a coherent information system. There is no silver bullet to resolve this problem, and detailed negotiations are required to achieve agreements with carriers. Some providers have indicated that these problems push them to change strategies and to link with what seems to be the most promising system at the time or with the carrier that best supports either the device that they plan to deploy or that most of their users have chosen on their own. These decisions are risky as no one knows which mDevice or carrier will be best in the future as new devices with new capabilities, as well as new carrier services and plans, are continuously evolving.

Considerations for mHealth

There are numerous considerations to be addressed in implementing mDevices in healthcare, including electromagnetic interference, authentication, data integrity, confidentiality, security, interoperability, brownouts, and clinical grade goals, as well as risk management, including managing multiple devices over multiple networks.

Electromagnetic Interference (EMI) and Electromagnetic Compatibility (EMC) within a Facility

In the late 1990s and early 2000s, it was recognized that cell phones may cause interruption and disruption of computerized medical devices through EMI. In response to concerns that EMI could be a serious problem resulting in patient harm, many hospitals and clinics issued policies forbidding the use of cell phones on their premises. Over time, as cell phones became better protected and caused less interference and as simple EMI management techniques were promulgated, these policies have been relaxed to one degree or another in most facilities. In any case, healthcare facilities should routinely have the potential impact of EMI assessed in their facilities.

Electromagnetic compatibility (EMC) "is the ability of electronic devices to coexist without adversely affecting their performance" (MoHCA 2004), and through the development of an EMC program, institutions can determine the extent to which cell phones may be used in their facilities. For instance, the proximity of a device and a cell phone is a major key for managing potential risks.

In general, the potential for EMI should not be taken lightly, but it also should be noted that both conducted EMI (for example, via wiring, AC) and radiated EMI (for example, via mDevices) can be of concern. Indeed, conducted EMI incidents are more common in clinical settings than are radiated ones, and few of the latter that cause adverse patient outcomes have been reported. This is due in part to existing technical and human safeguards that resolve an incident before it becomes critical. Even when serious malfunctioning of a medical device is identified, it often cannot be repeated under the same circumstances. Device malfunctioning is a complex event and may be caused partly by software, EMI, or other factors (MoHCA 2004).

Nevertheless, while interference is much reduced with modern cell phones and recent medical devices, it is still an issue with older medical devices and equipment and requires surveillance and compatibility management in any case. Not allowing any mDevices in clinical areas initially appeared to be the answer, but such a restriction results in the loss of clinically and administratively important benefits of mDevices. Further, enforcement of such a restriction may be difficult as the adoption and use of cell phones becomes increasingly pervasive. The best response to potential EMI is a well-designed EMC program that can mitigate EMI risk and facilitate adoption of mDevices, which in turn can reduce medical errors, improve the quality of care, and diminish costs (MoHCA 2004).

For more information on EMI and how to develop an effective EMC program, check FDA publications, rules, and guidelines regularly, as well as those of other relevant entities as they continue to address this issue.

Device Interoperability

Just as the goal with EMRs is to have them interoperable, users should be able to communicate with any kind of smartphone, cell phone, or PDA over any Wi-Fi, WLAN, broadband, or other network, as authorized and authenticated, independent of carrier, as well as with remote monitoring devices. The mobile industry is moving toward this goal of interoperability, and each healthcare institution has to ensure that it is achieved, to the greatest extent possible, within its environment.

The degree to which data transmitted from an mDevice can be readily integrated within the healthcare records of the receiver will vary, depending on the institution's progress toward EMR adoption; that is, EMRs are generally the limiting factor. mDevice-generated XML-based information enables most mDevices to communicate data with one another and with some EMRs, although limitations may result when an application is available on one type of device but not on another. However, some EMR systems, including some legacy systems, may not be able to accommodate XML-based data. In any case, those with EMRs should have the information transmitted and incorporated directly into the EMR, where possible, or into Web-based repositories that link to the EMR, or they can create PDFs or scanned documents out of the data and incorporate these into the EMR records. Of course, those providers who still function primarily with paper records will have to receive data transmitted from an mDevice by fax or electronically in the browsers of their computers and print out the documents for insertion into their paper records.

Clinical Grade mHealth

The term *clinical grade* has been coined to describe the requirements of mDevices and mobile systems in healthcare. Clinical grade systems provide the following:

- **24/7 availability**—Anytime, anyplace, anywhere, with back-up alternatives in the event of system failure.

- **Integrated security**—Dependability, information privacy, integrity and regulatory compliance (HIPAA, ARRA, FDA, and so on); only authenticated, logged access by authorized persons; networkwide layered defense model.

- **Quality of service (QofS) and guaranteed service level agreements (SLA)**—Consistent user experience, trusted service, solution risk-taking, measured traffic

- **Pervasive coverage of the facility and beyond**—Communication anywhere, anytime

- **Seamless mobility with session adaptation**—System accommodates any mobile device.

- **Transaction integrity**—System assures data cannot be altered during transactions.

- **Nonrepudiation**—Authentication can be proved to be genuine.

- **Ability to evolve**—Capabilities can expand without losing other clinical grade characteristics.

- **Human system interactions**—Ease and consistency of use

- **Workflow engagement**—Integrated into workflow to accelerate adoption, adapting on demand. (Graves et al. 2005) (Wallace and Graves 2006) (Beaulieu 2009)

Further, the service path of an end-to-end application should not exceed a downtime of three minutes per year (99.999 percent reliability), and the downtime for major application service should not be more than one minute per year (also close to 99.999 percent reliability). Similarly, the end user application failure rate should not exceed one incident per year (Beaulieu 2009).

It must be emphasized that at present these criteria should be viewed more as ideals or goals, than as requirements because few, if any, mobile installations meet them to their fullest degree. Equally important is the acknowledgment that these goals and mDevice capabilities far exceed the capabilities of today's EMR systems. Thus, we are setting the bar higher for mobile systems than we have set it for EMR systems, just as we have set higher expectations for EMRs than we have for paper records. Nevertheless, it is essential that health information managers work closely with their HIT colleagues to strive to achieve the goals of clinical grade mobile systems to the greatest extent possible, given the characteristics of the devices, services, systems, and the institution itself. It is also essential that HIM professionals apply these efforts and goals to EMRs as well. This includes communicating their expectations to both mobile and EMR system vendors. For more information on "clinical grade," follow the Web site links to the sources cited above.

Brownouts

A handful of hospitals reported in 2009 that they have approximately 10,000 wireless devices in operation within their campuses, leading to the fear of brownouts; that is, overuse of the transmission capabilities that would bring all their wireless communication to a standstill. Disaster plans, therefore, should address this potential. Standards committees, particularly IEEE, are addressing priority services for such situations.

Securing Wireless Transmissions

Information technology specialists, whether they are employees or contractors, have the primary technical responsibility for designing wireless systems and securing wireless transmissions. Nevertheless, it behooves the HIM professional to be informed about these technologies and of the decisions made and actions taken to achieve the expectations that the mobile systems will appropriately and adequately protect PHI. At the same time, HIM professionals should facilitate the utilization of mobile technologies, devices, and applications in order to maximize the delivery of good healthcare. Thus, HIM professionals must work closely with IT personnel, sharing their expertise and contributing to decisions related to the design and adoption of wireless systems in their facilities. General information that will assist HIM professionals in these roles is discussed next.

While there are several options for securing Wi-Fi networks, they are not equal or interchangeable. Static wired equivalent privacy (WEP) is an old standard that is interoperable with most wireless network devices. That interoperability makes it attractive, but it is not recommended for a number of reasons, including that it is easily cracked. While dynamic WEP is safer and more secure than static WEP, more advanced encryption options are available and should be used if at all possible. Wi-Fi protected access (WPA) is more secure than either form of WEP, and it is applicable on both personal and institutional networks, as is a more advanced and more secure version, WPA2. WPA2 is the government's standard for security, which makes it, at present, the preferred standard (Tewson and Riley 2008).

Improvements to wireless security will no doubt continue to evolve, as will their adoption in healthcare. The HIM professional should stay alert to these developments as well as to both realized and potential threats and, as noted previously, should work closely with IT personnel to assure their facility is adequately protecting PHI.

Encryption

Encryption transforms readable data into a form that lacks meaning and prevents it from being read. This requires use of a confidential process or key to revert it back to its readable form. A digital signature is a form of encryption that uniquely identifies and authenticates the sender of the message, but not the message itself.

Message encryption may be secret key or public key based. Secret keys are called symmetric because they involve the exchange of a secret key with the party to whom the encrypted message is being sent. It is cumbersome because the secret key must be sent before or after the message itself is sent, thus requiring two communications in place of one, and the key has limited use (once or for a limited period of time) because the receiver now knows the secret key.

Public key encryption, also called asymmetric key encryption is preferred. Public key encryption requires two keys, a public one and a private one. Only the public key can be used to encrypt a message, while only the private key can be used to decrypt it. Thus, the sender uses the receiver's public key to encrypt and send the message. A certificate authority (the key keeper, so to speak) validates the public key and allows the message to be decrypted with a one-time use private key so that the receiver knows it was not altered and, of course, can read it. Further, when the message being sent is signed with the sender's private key (a digital signature), the receiver can confirm that the message was sent by the person claiming to have sent it, thus authenticating the sender. Asymmetric key encryption, then, can be used both to confirm the sender or author of the message and to be assured the message has not been altered.

Authentication

Authentication is the unmistakable proof of who (or what) created the documentation and that this person or entity takes responsibility for the correctness of such data input (for example, with a wet or electronic signature). The goal is to apply standard healthcare documentation authentication requirements to mDevices. At any time after documentation, it should be possible to confidently identify not only who created an entry but also whether it was in draft mode or final mode with the originator's signature. This is done easily with handwritten and transcribed documents, but how can it be assured with an mDevice?

Authentication may be basic, certificate-based, or two-factor. Basic authentication requires that the client submit a user name and password, and the server, after verifying their validity, grants access to the client. It should be used only when secure socket layer (SSL) is enabled because this increases communication security between the client and server.

As noted previously in the section on encryption, certificate-based authentication uses digital certificates that uniquely identify individuals, enabling secure, confidential communication between them. The certificate authority (CA), again the key keeper that issues the certificates, acts as a third party that confirms the individuals' identities and assures that the certificates cannot be altered.

As the name implies, two-factor authentication has two parts. As described by John Parmigiani in a 2009 AHIMA webinar on the challenge of managing portable devices, it includes two of the following: something you know (typically a user ID, password, or PIN, but also a screen touch pattern unique to the user), something you have (for example, a token key, or badge), or something you are (such as a biometric ID—iris scan, fingerprint, voice scan). Touch patterns can be particularly appealing to users who then do not have to remember a series of numbers and/or letters. although with pattern recognition, they must remember the touch pattern that unlocks the device; but for some, the finger may remember touch patterns more readily than the mind remembers numbers and letters. Tokens, each with a unique serial number assigned to an individual, generate a unique number that changes minute by minute. This form of authentication typically requires the user to enter his user name and password (things he knows), and the unique number generated by the token (something he has) in order to gain access to the server. Some online banking services use token-based authentication, while others rely on certificate-based authentication.

mDevice users should use authentication to turn on the mDevice, but if the device belongs to the user, it may be difficult to enforce him or her doing so. More control can be exerted when the devices are provided by the institution, in which case the mDevice can be programmed to require authentication that identifies (authenticates) the user who unlocks it and includes timed auto log off. In any case, a separate log in for applications with patient-related information must be required, and here certificate-based or two-factor authentication is important, particularly when such applications link the user to the institution's virtual private network (VPN) and patient information. Further, if documentation is done on or through the mDevice, it also should record the time of documentation. Of course, it is advisable within a provider setting to have clinicians acknowledge that they are responsible for proper documentation, including authentication, no matter what mode they use, including mDevices. Again, it will be up to the IT personnel to address the technological aspects of such requirements, with HIM professionals assuring they are addressed, that they are enabled, that users are required to abide by them, and that adherence to these requirements is monitored. That also means users must document acknowledgment of these obligations.

No doubt it will be important for mDevices and applications to offer different kinds of identification systems so that users can choose what fits them best. Such is already the case with many mDevices, either with "out of the box" options or through add-on applications selected by the user to match his preference. Again, however, when access to patient data is involved, certificate-based or two-factor authentication should be required.

An interesting new development is mDevice identification. This method is based on agreements between clinicians and provider institutions that a certain mobile phone is used only by a specific user. That user takes responsibility for assuring that no one else uses the device and that he will take immediate action when the phone is lost, stolen, or malfunctioning. In such cases, an agreement can be documented that identifies all calls from this phone as coming from the assigned user, supplemented perhaps by voice recognition. It is important here to point out that voice recognition is not synonymous with speech recognition. Speech recognition engines are designed to recognize and transcribe or otherwise document the spoken word. Voice recognition is quite different in that it requires a system to compare the voice of the individual calling against the stored voice of the individual that caller is claiming to be. If there is a match, the user is authenticated.

Then there is the issue of synchronization of applications that are independent of the provider's health information system (HIS). These are applications that users may install on their mobile devices and that may include or link to patient information that is entered or accessed separately and apart from connections to the provider institution. Such information may come from the patient herself, from the provider's private practice, or from other sources, including potentially from the provider institution. To access such applications and the information they include, providers should set up authentication that will not allow others who have access to the device to also have access to these applications and their contents. This, of course, requires the application providers to design such applications so that they require separate and appropriate, strong authentication for access.

The ability of an institution to control which applications their providers use and the degree to which that provider's patient information is entered into these applications is limited. That is not to say that an institution cannot prohibit the use of such applications and/or the entering of patient data into them. But an individual provider's actions and practices may vary from an institution's policies, particularly when the provider believes, correctly or incorrectly that such applications aid in treating the patients relevant to them. Consider, for example, disease management applications, where the ability to monitor a diabetic patient's blood sugar could enhance that patient's day-to-day diet and exercise and, therefore, help control of her diabetes. What is within the institution's control, however, is to require that providers have the patient's authorization for entering, storing, and accessing PHI in mDevices and in their applications and that the provider acknowledges his responsibility to assure protection of PHI and to meet the regulatory and institutional requirements for doing so.

Data Integrity

Just as with more traditional modes of documentation, data integrity requires that recorded information cannot be changed once it is in final form; that is, once it has been signed/authenticated. If changes and/or corrections subsequently are made, they must be properly labeled as such, they must identify who amended what and when it was amended, and they must provide access to the original entry that was changed or corrected. Data integrity on mDevices can be ensured with digital signatures and audit logs so that data entries are signed off on digitally and access to data is recorded in logs that identify who accessed what, when it was accessed, and what, if anything, was changed. As in paper records, changes and corrections will inevitably occur. The goal is not to restrict these changes but to require that they are recorded in a manner that assures they are recognizable and retrievable, just as they are in paper records and should be in EMRs.

An agreement should be reached with users that when a communication is sent for entry into a patient's record, it must have been authenticated so that it cannot be amended in any way. Exceptions are communications clearly labeled as drafts. Amendments to authenticated entries must be done in a new communication, and the HIM department must carefully manage such amendments by linking them to the original. Further, the system must assure that information cannot be discarded or changed without leaving an audit trail. These data integrity features may be as difficult to implement with mDevices as they are with EMRs. So, just as more and more EMR vendors are addressing this gap in their systems, so must mDevice and applications providers. The much wider adoption of mDevices may be a greater incentive to vendors to achieve the requirements of data integrity so that they are more competitive in an increasingly competitive environment of mHealth.

Synchronization of Patient Information

As with EMRs (and paper records, for that matter), it will be difficult with mDevices to assure that the system accesses the most current information and that additional repositories within the information system are updated with that latest information. It will be more difficult to assure this with mHealth systems than with EMRs. Information can be downloaded onto a storage card within the mDevice, leading to the potential of several parallel storage sites (for example, the EMR system at the provider site, the "summarized" record [such as a CCR record in a site such as Google Health], and the data stored on the mDevice. HIM and HIT professionals must be alert to such scenarios and must assure that synchronization for such occasions is addressed within the provider institution's IT strategies.

Security Considerations and Concerns of Managing Data Across Multiple Devices and Networks

Multiple device and network management, with an emphasis on security, is a growing concern in all industries, and it is of particular concern in healthcare, given the demands and requirements related to protection of PHI. Todd Crick of inCode proposes five Cs for designing and managing a secure connectivity platform for machine to machine (M2M; also mobile to mobile) to address concerns for connectivity, device management, identity management, and security. In brief, Crick's five Cs are (Crick 2009):

- *Configuration*, which includes the ability to remotely activate and provision devices, conduct device diagnostics and diagnostics on antivirus software and firewall protection, upgrade and manage the firmware (programs that internally control the devices), and distribute and upgrade applications.

- *Connectivity*, which includes automatically detecting and managing devices, preselecting and preconnecting to the best available network, activating or deactivating individual or multiple devices, securing access to corporate networks for remote users and devices, and monitoring key network performance indicators.

- *Control*, which includes managing user authentication and passwords, transmitting data securely (encryption and data integrity), backing up content on devices over-the-air (OTA), locking and unlocking devices OTA, wiping devices when they are lost or stolen, and managing identity for multiple use profiles.

- *Convenience*, which includes single click user sign on, self care of devices by end users, Web services that integrate with portals to "My Account" (for example, for PHRs), and customized reporting for audits and operation management.

- *Content*, which includes storing content across multiple devices (for example, digital vault), content access and management across multiple devices, and integrated services across multiple devices and networks.

While the technological responsibility for achieving the goals of the security program will fall to IT specialists, the HIM professional must be a part of the team that identifies the expectations and designs, administers the security system, and monitors security management of PHI.

Limitations of mDevices

The limits of mDevices include size, readability, keyboard or touch screen entry, the level of connectivity, battery life, storage capacity, and review and editing vulnerabilities. For decades, advocates of computers and new technical devices claimed that technology will automatically provide safer care and reduce errors in documentation and decision-making. The example of illegible hand writing is often cited as a weakness of paper records, while computer entry is touted as more correct and/or more precise. A more balanced view shows that users can make at least as many mistakes with a computer as they can with traditional documentation systems. A clinician easily could type the wrong key on a device. If such a mistake involved the wrong dosage with a misplaced decimal, the results could be grave.

Or imagine if all of the clinicians in an organization are using mDevices and they find that, for one reason or another, they do not have connectivity. For those clinicians, the whole care system may collapse. Even more likely is the occasional problem of a clinician stepping outside the range of service and losing connectivity and perhaps all data as well. Quality of service (QoS) for mHealth systems is an essential priority when planning and installing systems.

Synchronization of data captured from medical devices and mDevices is a major concern for the biomedical engineering department, and HIM professionals must coordinate with them to assure not only the ability but also the accuracy and audit trail of such synchronization.

Misuse and loss is another concern. Policies must require that clinicians not allow others to use any mDevice they use to access, store, or record patient information, and that clinicians are aware of the ramifications of not adhering to such policies. If a clinician who uses his mDevice for prescribing allows his daughter to use the device to contact friends, there is not only the potential breach of confidentiality through her accessing confidential patient information but also the risk of her using the prescribing system to access drugs for her or her friends. mDevices get lost, stolen, or damaged all the time. It is important to emphasize the need to destroy all the data remotely when a device is lost or stolen and to be informed of both the loss of the device and confirmation that its content has been destroyed, including documentation of same. Synchronization between the old and the new devices also should be regulated.

A provider institution must alert clinicians to the importance of review and editing. Traditionally, an entry could be dictated and the physician would rely on the medical transcriptionist to edit it as necessary for clarity, accuracy, and completeness. Then, after transcription, the clinician would have an opportunity to review and edit the text further, if appropriate, before signing it. This may not be the case with mDevices. Many offer "auto-complete" (as letters are entered, the systems suggest word completion) and "auto-signature" (systems that do not require or encourage review of a clinical note or other documentation prior to its authentication). Clinicians must understand the new and potentially dangerous consequences of such functionalities, and institutions must guard against them.

Outdated Technologies and Merging Legacy Systems

The capabilities of mDevices are exploding. Using a cell phone that is more than a year or two old may be limiting and potentially problematic. Biomedical engineers, for example, may be legitimately concerned that older phones (perhaps five years or older) may cause interference with medical devices that newer phones would not. This is another reason why HIM or HIT professionals should maintain an inventory of the devices used by those affiliated with their institution. Further, healthcare institutions may consider encouraging clinicians to replace old devices every 12 to 18 months, or the institution itself may choose to underwrite their doing so.

Much more challenging is the integration into legacy systems. Most provider information systems are proprietary, with some systems having developed more options for mDevice integration than others. Currently it is not clear if and when the majority of providers will implement systems that allow easier integration of mobile computing and communication systems as well as easier interoperability with other EMR systems. This is a complicated issue that touches many related topics and developments, including the transition from messaging standards to Internet XML.

Selecting Devices and Applications

Usability and user friendliness are essential in selecting mDevices and their applications, and because user preferences differ, the devices are most likely to be used successfully if users select their own devices. Patients choose their own devices, and clinicians have some choice. However, there are instances where an institution will adopt a systemwide device, in which case, the institution will likely take on the burden of financing them. Whether the end user makes the selection or not, there are several factors to consider in assessing the choices for mHealth devices and applications in order to achieve successful implementation.

Regarding the device itself, screen size is important, although the larger the size, the larger and potentially the heavier the unit, which is another important factor. Orientation of the screen is also a consideration—portrait, landscape, or both. Clarity of screen image varies among devices, as does the choice (or not) of screen wallpaper and colors and selecting what information and applications will routinely appear on the opening screen. Keyboard options also must be taken into consideration. Is the keyboard separate from the screen? If so, consider its size, visibility, and the touch of its keys. Is it a standard keyboard or a numeric one, requiring multiple taps on a number to enter letters? For on-screen touch keyboards, size, visibility, and touch are also important, especially in relationship to the user's finger size and touch or sensitivity. With any kind of keyboard, does it offer auto-complete? This can be both a strength and a weakness. For routine, nonclinical use, it is very helpful. For clinical uses, it can lead to potentially dangerous errors. Battery life, too, is important, but this can be difficult to assess; talk-time battery life may differ greatly from Web access or application-specific battery life, and of course the usage patterns of individuals vary greatly. Storage capacity, too, must be considered; the potential number and size of applications will vary from device to device as will the needs and preferences of one user to another. One of the most important factors to assess is navigation. How do users sign-on? How do users choose and open an application? How do users move from application to application? Does the system allow multiple applications to be open at once? These are just some of the questions to explore. Ease of navigation can be critical: the simpler and the more intuitive, the better.

Choosing a device may mean choosing among carriers that support the device or may require accepting the unique carrier to which it is linked. In either case, carrier plans that are required or offered must be assessed. Monthly costs, usage plans and associated costs, data versus voice costs, text messaging costs, Internet access costs, international usage costs, and required term (time) of contract are among the important considerations. Of course, when the institution is choosing devices for some or all of its personnel, discounts are in order and must be compared and negotiated. It is possible, too, that in instances where the institution does not supply or require a particular device, one or more device manufacturers (or a carriers) may offer discounts to employees and contractors affiliated with an institution, in which case negotiations also come into play.

Institutions considering providing devices for some or all of their clinicians and other staff, also may want to consider engaging contract services that will guide them through the selection, procurement, deployment training, implementation, 24/7 ongoing monitoring, technical advice, security, repair, maintenance, and replacement, of their mHealth rollout.

The range of applications to choose from varies from device to device, so this also is important. However, selection doesn't end with knowing which applications are offered, because the applications themselves must be compared and assessed. The following principles regarding application usability are recommended by Hal Miller-Jacobs (2009) for mDevice application developers. (The recommendations have been modified here to guide potential buyers in their selection process.)

- **Design**—Screen design and information displays should fit the limited real estate and the user's activity level.

- **Screen usage**—Screen and information displays should eliminate the extraneous and include the essential. The ability to zoom in and out can enhance visibility and usability, making it an attractive feature, provided that it is simple to do.

- **Display format and device orientation**—The display of information should match the width of the screen (portrait or landscape orientation), and when both orientations are available in the same device, it should auto adjust as the user moves between them.

- **User needs**—The user should be comfortable with each phase of the application. Options can be important. For example, documentation options could include speech, keyboard, and touch screen, with the user selecting among them according to the type of data to be entered—numeric, textual, line-drawing.

- **Screen reloads**—Applications should offer direct links and shortcuts to the greatest extent possible to avoid long reloads.

- **Auto-complete**—Avoid auto-complete options in medical applications that may lead to inaccurate and potentially dangerous entries. (Note: This can be difficult to achieve with mDevice applications, just as it is with EMRs. However, some medical application developers either do not offer auto-complete or do not allow the user to turn it off.)

- **Clear feedback**—Screen highlighting of choices made can help reduce medical errors. Requiring confirmation for critical decisions is also advised in this regard.

- **Browser controls**—Generally, on-screen navigation controls, such as back, forward, and cancel, can facilitate use if they are simple to use. Whether on-screen or off, such controls should not frustrate the user by slow or poor responsiveness.

- **Test, retest, and retest**—Seek trial usage whenever possible.

Of course, cost is important regarding both devices and applications. Finally, research is essential. Read about them online, on the vendor's Web sites, in comparison studies, in user blogs, and on social networks. Find current users in your institution or community. The research also should include test driving them before buying them, in simulations online and/or in stores. All such research is important.

CHAPTER 5

Best Practices

Introduction

The rise of mDevices requires HIM professionals to implement new systems and policies to assure their legality and that professionals within the organization use them according to those policies. For decades, health information professionals have guided and guarded the healthcare processes of information capture, storage, and transmission, even when such systems were purely paper based. The digitization of information through the computer has now provided a new challenge as systems move from handwriting to computer input and from dictation and transcription to speech recognition and direct input. It is challenging for clinicians to work with a desktop computer and type entries into the EMR. Using mDevices is even more challenging. There is a learning process associated with using a touch-screen keyboard on a unit such as the Android or iPhone. What safeguards must HIM implement? If an organization faces legal challenges years later, how can it testify to the authentication of such devices?

More complex is the issue of transmission. Is it possible in an organization's wireless system for a physician to think she sent a message, but due to lack of coverage, the message is lost? Is a copy retained on the device or elsewhere? Is a copy automatically sent to the HIM department? Has the system been set up so the department can monitor the sending and receipt of messages? What resources are needed for such monitoring? Of the many issues related to mHealth, the need to safeguard protected health information (PHI) is a priority.

Risk Management of mDevice Security

Risks related to mDevices increase when there is increased connectivity, a greater number of devices, and an increased number of applications on those devices. The value of the content to be protected (in this case, PHI) and the value of the devices are other factors that increase the risk. In contrast, the risk is decreased when software is removed from the system and/or device, the number of users is decreased, user privileges are removed or limited, use of the system is reduced, and the value of the system itself is reduced (Lindstrom 2009). However, these limitation techniques need to be balanced against the value of the devices and the information on them in terms of their impact on patient care. So an organization needs to exert control but should not go to extremes. For example, a no cell phone policy not only eliminates the potential benefits of anywhere, anytime communication on healthcare delivery and institutional productivity but also could negatively impact relationships between the organization, its clinicians, its employees, and even its patients. So risk management becomes a balancing act.

Smartphone risk management requires protecting against data loss. This includes requiring secure passwords and timeouts with automatic locking of devices after a specified period of nonuse. There also must be encryption of data at rest and in transit, and, of course, the device must be remotely wiped if it is lost or stolen. Further, synching of institutional e-mail should be restricted to compliant devices only.

Protection against malware includes implementing application controls that can restrict certain applications from being installed, restricting port usage to approved ports (a Web point of access to aggregated information, such as a patient portal to PHRs), and enabling only authorized input/output capabilities (for example, Infrared, Wi-Fi). Other organizational challenges related to mDevices include the blurred distinction between enterprise devices and consumer devices, with many devices being used for both professional and personal needs and executives (and in the healthcare world, clinicians) driving adoption of mDevices, which IT (and in healthcare, HIM) must accommodate and manage. Further complicating matters, there are multiple competing platforms in the mobile world, as no operating system (OS) system (for example, Windows Mobile, Symbian, and Linux) is dominant, thus requiring management of not only multiple devices but also multiple networks (Gow 2009).

Data Safeguarding Solutions

Safeguarding data against security threats, whether at rest or in transmission, requires 24/7 security monitoring by either in-house or contract services. This includes vulnerability and breach detection and prevention, with appropriate administrators and other personnel being notified immediately of such detections and advising them of response efforts and resolution.

Because wireless connections are ubiquitous these days, but not all such connections are secure, vulnerabilities are rampant, particularly in public places such as coffee shops, libraries, and even public areas in healthcare institutions, such as waiting rooms, where wireless connectivity is available to patients and visitors. Likewise, the utilization of wireless devices by clinicians, employees, and contractors is widespread, and many of these may use their mDevices over insecure networks. Consequently, the potential exposure to data theft is widespread on cell phones, laptops, e-mail and Web mail, Twitter and similar social networking sites, text messaging, instant messaging, USB drives and other portable storage media, as well as any unsecured communications.

Certainly HIPAA, the American Recovery and Reinvestment Act (ARRA), state, and other regulations, as well as institutional policies and procedures, must be addressed and their requirements must be met not only to protect PHI but also to protect the institution against the consequences of data theft. Thus, sound security policies and procedures must be developed, disseminated, acknowledged, adhered to, and monitored in order to avoid the likelihood of data loss as well as its consequences, which not only include potential damage to the patient but also high financial costs through penalties and damage control, as well as damage to the institution's reputation. Prevention is much less costly all around.

Already existing PHI security measures must be extended to assure they meet the potential threats associated with mDevices. These include viruses, malware, hackers, RFID, applications, Bluetooth, unapproved downloading and storage of PHI, and unsecured networks as noted previously.

Whether the devices are owned by the healthcare organization or by users employed or otherwise affiliated with the institution, if they are being used to access, hold, or transmit PHI that is under the stewardship of the institution, their use must be monitored. That includes cataloging them, including what devices are being used by whom (and their access rights and privileges), for what purpose, where (on campus and/or off), and with what applications (including their versions) installed on them that are designed for or may be used to access, store, or transmit PHI and what data security measures exist in relationship to the device and the data itself. Additionally, network connections can be remotely monitored to assure compliance with PHI-related and other organizational policies.

Data Threats

We will address medical identify theft briefly and then give greater attention to PHI theft.

Medical Identity Theft

According to AHIMA's e-HIM Work Group on Medical Identify Theft (2008), "Medical identity theft is the inappropriate or unauthorized misrepresentation of individually identifiable health information for the purpose of obtaining access to property or services, which may result in long-lasting harm to an individual interacting with the healthcare continuum." It goes on to explain that this may be to access healthcare services for which they are not eligible or perhaps to obtain illegal or otherwise unattainable drugs for themselves or others. Such thefts can be costly to the provider and provider institution, the patient whose identity has been stolen, the payer, and society in general. The practice brief gives important guidance for a risk analysis, as well as measures for prevention and detection and responding to instances of medical identify theft, and it is reprinted in the appendices of this document.

The potential vulnerability of mDevices to medical identity theft requires particular attention to accurately identifying patients who are using such devices to request or access healthcare services. Secure user names and passwords to access the institution's portal play an important role, and of course, it is important that the patient's authorization to communicate their health information through mobile communications—voice, e-mail, text messaging, Web browsers—be documented. Actually, mobile communications offer the potential for greater safeguards to patient identity than do "traditional" phone communications, where often a name, birth date, and perhaps address and telephone number may be the extent to which patient identification is assured.

PHI Data Theft

HIM professionals must work closely with legal counsel and IT personnel to guard against data theft, in particular that of PHI, through the establishment and implementation of appropriate policies related to privacy, security, and compliance with federal regulations such as HIPAA and ARRA, state regulations, and accreditation guidelines. As noted earlier, two-factor security is preferred for interconnectivity, and all data should be secured through encryption. An educational program for all personnel with access to patient data is essential, both when an individual initiates employment or a contract relationship with the organization and periodically (at least annually) thereafter, and whenever there are changes to requirements or their implementation. The HIM professional should also assure that appropriate insurance coverage is in place in the event of a data theft but should not regard such coverage as a protection against less-than-adequate, recommended or required measures to protect against data theft (Wernick 2007).

Safeguarding Data

We will now turn to how to safeguard against such threats. Measures include device tracking and loss prevention, as well as clearing the memory.

Device Tracking and Loss Prevention

GPS location systems are useful not only in the event a device needs memory clearance but also to track devices that the institution owns, leases, or is otherwise responsible for. Again, applications are available that can locate a device and, for that matter, its user. The latter ability raises legitimate concerns about privacy. If you know where my device is, you know where I am, unless the device is misplaced, lost, or stolen, or I have chosen not to have it with me or have disabled that function. This applies to providers, employers, contractors, and patients. So the capacity to use device tracking for devices under the control of the institution (for example, those they lease or own and grant the use of to providers, patients, and employees) must be communicated to such users, who by virtue of accepting and using them authorize that they be tracked. Documentation of the same is best done by a formal agreement. In the case of an institution using GPS location systems to track devices that they do not own or lease, the institution must document such tracking by authorization of the user with specification of when such tracking will be done (for example, in case of emergency or disaster).

Device tracking also may be used for equipment, supplies, and paper medical records, as addressed earlier, where RFID for example can help to control and maintain the institutional inventory of such items. Of course, such use for patient tracking must be legitimate and authorized.

Clearing the Memory

In the event an mDevice is lost or stolen, or the user knows its security has been compromised, it should be possible to clear the device's memory remotely. Most mDevice instruction manuals give directions on how to clear the memory when the device is in hand. Additionally, remote memory clearance may be offered by the device manufacturer or carrier or through an application downloaded to the device. Remote clearance is done through the Internet, which, through a global positioning system (GPS), accesses the device and related application and erases the memory. While the procedures may be generally similar from device to device, carrier to carrier, or application to application, they likely differ in specifics. Whether memory clearance applies to all content on the device or to specific applications will also vary across devices. Of course, memory should be cleared as well when a device or application is no longer being used or is replaced, or when the device is passed on to the next user (for example, when the devices are supplied by the institution and moved from resident to resident during residency rotations).

The HIM professional (or the IT department, depending on institutional policy) should maintain documentation regarding memory clearance procedures for at least the more commonly used devices, but it will be impossible to be aware of all the different devices and applications in use and their current version. Such information should be available through device, carrier, and application Web sites, where earlier versions likely will be accessible as well.

When the HIM professional becomes aware of the need to clear a device's memory, he should immediately contact the user (or the IT specialist responsible for this process), explain the situation, and direct that the memory be cleared. Of course, if it is the user who first becomes aware of the need to clear memory, she must do so and notify the HIM and/or IT department. In all instances, appropriate personnel, according to the policies and practices of the institution, should also be notified. If security of PHI has been breached, the patient or patients in question should also be notified, according to institutional procedures and HIPAA, ARRA, and state requirements.

Breaches Involving PHI

The American Recovery and Reinvestment Act of 2009 amends HIPAA requirements regarding breach provisions applying to covered entities and business associates. In a recent AHIMA blog, Peter Adler, an attorney at law, reviewed these breach notification requirements following an unauthorized acquisition, access, use, or disclosure of unsecured (that is, unencrypted) PHI that compromises the security or privacy of such information. Notification must be made without reasonable delay after discovery of the breach and no later than 60 days following such discovery. HIPAA and ARRA regulations apply to electronic as well as paper-based PHI, and thus they apply to PHI stored or accessed or transmitted through mDevices as well. HIM professionals must stay alert to revised and new requirements regarding breach provisions, as this is a dynamic environment.

Notification by a covered entity to each individual whose unsecured PHI has been breached must include the following:

- "what happened, including the date of the breach and the date of the discovery of the breach, if known; the types of unsecured PHI that were involved in the breach (such as full name, Social Security number, date of birth, home address, account number, or disability code); steps that may be taken by individuals to protect themselves from potential harm resulting from the breach;

- what the covered entity involved is doing to investigate the breach, to mitigate losses, and to protect against any further breaches; and

- procedures for individuals to ask questions or learn additional information, which shall include a toll-free telephone number and e-mail address, Web site, or postal address" (Adler 2009).

When the breach of PHI involves a business associate, notification to the covered entity of the breach must identify each individual whose PHI was, or is reasonably believed to have been, accessed, acquired, or disclosed by the business associate during the breach (Adler 2009).

Thus, HIM professionals responsible for PHI in covered entities must have policies and procedures in place not only to address breaches by the covered entity itself but also by its business associates and must have signed agreements with such business associates delineating and requiring them to acknowledge their responsibilities regarding PHI and notification of its breach.

In this new world, providers must be advised of and required to comply with PHI policies, yet many provider institutions have not yet fully adjusted to the legal requirements related to EMRs. Wireless communication adds a major layer to such responsibilities and efforts. If policies are not appropriately established and implemented, a provider may be sitting on a legal time bomb.

Among those policies should be a data breach notification response plan that (1) identifies which systems store data (know where your data are), (2) identifies who is on the response team (which should include representatives from HIM and IT, legal/compliance, and communications/PR and perhaps others), (3) specifies the different federal and state requirements (which differ widely), (4) assures contracts with third parties that require them to provide immediate notice in the event of a breach, and (5) includes data breach insurance coverage (Sabett 2009).

Physician, Employee, and Contractor Responsibilities and Training

Health information and IT professionals must work with both internal and external users when it comes to the use of mDevices in healthcare. While there are similarities and overlaps regarding responsibilities and training of both groups, there are sufficient differences to warrant addressing them separately.

Internal Users

Adoption of mDevices by patient care providers is accelerating. Physicians use them to access, record, and transmit patient information at the point of care and remotely—patient information housed both in their practices and in the provider institutions where they have privileges, limited of course to each institution's ability and willingness to allow such access and the restrictions surrounding such use. Providers also are increasingly using mDevices for direct patient communications by e-mail and text message (as well as voice, of course) and for disease management, both by receiving monitored data from patients (for example, blood pressure and blood glucose) and by advising patients and reminding them of appointments and tests. The mDevice also provides remote and point-of-care access to resources such as formularies, guidelines, and protocols. Increasing numbers of physicians are using these devices for applications in each of the 12 clusters outlined in Chapter 2.

Nurses also frequently use mDevices, and it is anticipated that their use will continue to expand. Nurses are mobile in their jobs. According to a recent study, nurses walk an average of three miles per day (some up to five miles) on the job. They spend 31 percent of their shifts in patients' rooms, 38 percent at the nurses station, 24 percent on the unit, and 7 percent off the unit. They spend 35 percent of their time documenting patient care, doing so only 3 percent of the time in patients' rooms, 81 percent of the time at the nurses station, and the remainder elsewhere on or off the unit (Hendrich, Chow, Skiercynzki, and Zhengqiang 2008). Enabling nurses to record observations and vital signs at patients' bedsides increases the time that they spend with patients rather than going back and forth between patient rooms and the nurses station to do so.

Both clinicians and pharmacists are using mobile phones to consult formularies, check for adverse drug reactions, document intervention, and confirm insurance coverage. Other patient care providers also are increasing their use of mDevices for patient communications, documentation, access to resources, monitoring, and more.

The proliferation of healthcare-related applications is growing into the thousands. Many relate to patient-provider communications, and many are specific to provider needs, putting guidelines, protocols, formularies, and other expert resources literally at providers' fingertips. Even those specific to patient use are impacting the healthcare delivery system because patients are referencing information gained through online searches (about themselves in particular as well as about healthcare in general) in communications with their healthcare providers. Additionally, it is the healthcare provider herself who alerts the patient to the value of one or more of these applications, and such communications also come through educational programs put on by the healthcare institution. The HIM professional has an opportunity here to work with clinicians to develop and promote an online library of resources for both patients and clinicians.

Regarding providers' online access to patient information, such access must be limited to those patients for whom the providers have responsibility and authorized access. It is the responsibility of HIM and IT personnel to work cooperatively to establish policies that clearly delineate who has rights of access to what patient information and to assure that the HIM and IT systems reflect those policies and assure their effective administration. This must include not only restricting access where appropriate but also facilitating access where authorized. It also requires audit trails documenting who accessed what and when, restricting unauthorized access, and creating alerts when unauthorized access is attempted or achieved.

Internal mDevice users also include privacy and security officers, corporate information officers, and IT officers as well as department heads and their staff, including those in the HIM department. It is anticipated that more and more institutional personnel will become mDevice users both internally and externally to streamline their work, to enhance access, and to better support patient care delivery. Their access to PHI, of course, should be limited at least to the same extent such access is limited to paper and electronic medical records, with authorization, authentication, and audit trails required. The trend is toward controlling data elements rather than the whole medical record or even an entire document. As new technologies allow this, the provider system should be modified to allow data to be controlled in element sections.

External Users

Patient care providers also may be external users with authority to access information about patients for whom they are responsible. These may be providers whose patients have been admitted to the provider institution and who use mDevices to monitor their care, not only during their in-house visits but also through remote communications when back at their practice or elsewhere. Where hospitalists take over inpatient care, it is increasingly likely that external providers and the hospitalists and others treating patients in house will be in communication via mDevices.

Whatever the relationship between the external providers and the institution and its patients, in-house providers, and others, authorized communications about those patients should be facilitated at the same time that adequate controls are in place to assure the security of the communications and that documentation of such access is controlled, recorded, and monitored through appropriate authorization, authentication, and audit trails.

In selecting IT contractors, it is essential to assure that they have the qualifications to meet the expectations of the work they are engaged to do. Additionally, they must be required to document their understanding and agreement to the policies related to protection of institutional and patient information. The latter should be restricted so that IT contractors (and for that matter IT employees) do not have unnecessary access to patient information. However, there may be circumstances when the IT contractor unavoidably or unintentionally does have such access, and so their knowledge and acceptance of responsibility for protecting PHI is important. Since much of IT work, by its very nature, has to do with designing and managing security of medical records, this knowledge and commitment should be part and parcel of their competencies and obligations, supplemented by appropriate documentation of the same.

User Authorization and Authentication Controls

Anyone accessing PHI must be authorized to do so. Thus, system access must be designed to require user authentication and confirmation of this authorization before access is granted. Access rights, therefore, must be clearly defined and communicated to each potential user and nonuser within and outside the facility. Further, limitations and restrictions must be designed in such a way that access can be totally restricted, totally allowed, allowed only to certain parts of or data within the patient's record (for example, excluding behavioral information), allowed only in certain circumstances (for example, only during a particular episode of care when a provider is a consultant for a particular patient), and restricted to certain parts of the record (for example, restricting a dentist from patient information unrelated to the condition he is treating). Of course, the system must also allow "breaking the glass" so that in emergency circumstances, emergency personnel may access the record in order to know relevant patient healthcare status and treatment. Authentication of users in all of these instances must follow federal and state laws and regulations as well as institutional policies and procedures regarding PHI.

All clinicians, employees, and contractors who routinely, occasionally, or potentially have access to PHI, must be advised of and accept responsibility for safeguarding PHI in every way possible. Ongoing training is important and must occur upon employment or initial affiliation with the institution, with frequent reminders and updates as necessary. Training should address what the risks are to patients, the institution, the employee, the physician, and the contractor. Additionally, understanding of and acknowledgement of their responsibilities should be documented and updated regularly as well as on an ad hoc basis when circumstances warrant (for example, when policies themselves are updated). A recent AHIMA webinar emphasized some best practices that should be communicated to and required of mDevice users who have access to PHI through mDevices (Parmigiani 2009):

- Delete unnecessary information, keeping only what is needed for that day's activity on the device.

- Do not share devices that hold PHI.

- Notify the institution immediately if there is a loss or breach of PHI.

- Disable unneeded functions, including Bluetooth discoverable mode and 802.11 wireless when the device is not in use.

Off-campus Use of mDevices

All of the above requirements apply not just when the user is in house but also when mDevices are used off campus. And since many devices will be used both internally and externally, users must be vigilant in protecting PHI wherever they are, including when they are traveling. Special consideration must be given to instances when the user travels beyond U.S. borders. International travel is very different than interstate travel in that Fourth Amendment protections against search and seizure do not apply at U.S. borders, where border officials do not need probable cause, reasonable suspicion, or a warrant to seize laptops, smartphones, and other mDevices, including peripherals such as USB drives. Thus, the reasonable expectation of privacy does not apply, and these mDevices can be both searched and seized, putting PHI and other sensitive data at risk. Policies regarding travel with mDevices that can access or store PHI require special attention. Recommended tactics include using scrubbed devices made available in a loaner pool and leaving behind devices with PHI and other sensitive data. In any case, sensitive data should be left behind when traveling internationally, encryption must be enforced, and any breaches must be immediately reported to the organization. Should devices with sensitive data be seized at the border or sensitive data on them accessed, the notification and action plan should immediately involve legal counsel to determine appropriate action (Sabett 2009). It should be noted too that U.S. law does not apply outside the United States, giving even more reason for taking special precautions when traveling outside U.S. borders.

Policies, Procedures, and Security Agreements

The institution should have policies and procedures, as well as security agreements, in place, both to protect PHI and to document their efforts to do so. These should include requirements for:

- Device access control— Devices with access to PHI should be used only by the designated and authorized user. In instances where devices are supplied by the institution, a check-in/check-out procedure should be instituted, requiring devices to be signed in and out by the user. The device should be backed up and scanned for malware prior to check out and again upon check in, with periodic updates when assigned to a single user over an extended time (Dinh 2009).

- Access rights—Who is authorized to access what information under what circumstances?

- Authentication—Assuring that access is limited to those who can authenticate themselves to the system

- Multi-level passwords—For power-on, for exiting screen-savers, for accessing applications that include PHI, for connecting to networks that will give access to PHI. This, in particular, means for accessing the healthcare organization's network.

- Control of devices lost, stolen, no longer in use, or no longer authorized to be in use by clearing their memory, on site or remotely.

- Auditing use of devices, access to PHI, use of applications that can access, store, or transmit PHI.

- Using secure networks to store, access, and transmit PHI.

- Requiring and enforcing device and application locking (AirMagnet 2009).

Also important is to assure that the institution's disaster control procedures address mDevice use. It is quite likely, for example, that the use of mDevices in disaster situations will facilitate communications and delivery of care. Thus, the maintenance of a master list of contact information for all personnel, including mobile (and landline) phone numbers and e-mail (and street/city) addresses, is essential, with updates as reported but also with periodic prompts to all personnel to confirm or update current information. In the event of a disaster that requires immediate contact with all or some personnel, mass e-mails and text messages can be sent, with voice communications supplementing as necessary.

On the more negative side, institutions also must consider what to do in the event of a brownout—the overuse of transmission capabilities, leading to a wireless communications standstill. As noted previously, standards groups are addressing this, and both HIM and IT professionals should stay alert to their recommendations. Meanwhile, IT personnel should monitor the capacity and utilization of wireless communications to attempt to assure that the former stays well ahead of the latter. While not directly responsible for this technical requirement, the HIM director should be in regular communication with IT personnel and should be kept aware of both current and projected capacity and utilization patterns.

See Appendix A for some sample institutional policies and procedures, as well as a sample security agreement.

CHAPTER 6

Future Outlook of Portable Communication and Computing Devices

Introduction

Years ago, when two-way wireless communication was used mainly by law enforcement personnel or truckers to communicate with each other on the road, few would have anticipated that an advanced version of wireless communication would dramatically change the lives of people in the 21st century as dramatically as automobiles did in the 20th century. The first change wrought by mDevices was placing a powerful voice communication device into the hands of anyone just about anywhere, meaning people could call for help or simply stay in touch at anytime and were no longer tethered to their landline phone at home, work, or elsewhere. The second change offered nonvoice communication (that is, text messaging and e-mail), across not only communities and state lines but also across countries and oceans. The third change was the transformation of mobile devices into extensions of the Internet through powerful browsers. The fourth change is the increasingly expanding computing capabilities of such devices, making them location trackers, sports activity monitors, vital sign monitors disease managers, and so much more, thereby changing how we live and communicate. Just a few years ago, it was unthinkable that a mobile phone would be as important as a wallet to most people. Now it can be a person's multimedia communication device as well as an Internet browser, banking device, camera, portable music player, personal instructor, and more.

As we begin a new decade, mDevices have become an even more powerful information tool than the personal computer; some consumers are seeking desktop computers with the power and features of their iPhone or cell phone. There are tens of thousands of mDevice applications with that many and more anticipated. mDevices themselves are proliferating, and it is impossible to foresee which applications and devices will outpace today's favorites, never mind tomorrow's. Additionally, these devices continue to become easier to use, making them even more powerful. After centuries in which the smartest child was the one who could memorize the most, now the child who understands the big picture and is able to navigate through the wealth of information at her fingertips to find the right information is the smartest.

Several trends have been identified, but within each trend, the potential for innovation and surprise is vast.

What was once a wireless telephone for voice communication has already become a personal computer that is changing both knowledge and behavior, connecting anyone to a wealth of resources and information. Connectivity will reach the most remote village. This was unthinkable just a few decades ago.

The Future of mDevices in Healthcare

The impact of mDevices on healthcare and its stakeholders continues to spread. Today's mDevices prompt patients to take their medication on time, monitor patients' blood pressure, give providers access to guidelines, and offer real-time eligibility determination by payers, to name just a few of the thousands of mobile applications already available to the various stakeholders in healthcare.

Professional knowledge will be available in little applets to anyone who is able to use them. This will neutralize many of the privileges that were previously available only to professionals who in the past were the guardians of the scientific body of knowledge of their profession and controlled access to it. It will affect the hierarchy of healthcare because health information will be more accessible to and usable by patients and other nonclinicians, and there will be a "rethinking" of caregiver roles. Just as there will be consulting clinicians, concierge clinicians, Internet clinicians, coaching clinicians, and other new roles for clinicians, there also will be nonclinicians who will take on some of the traditional roles of the clinician. Think of the patient coach, helping patients understand their health status and problems and guiding them to digital and other resources; this is just one role that is emerging as a result of knowledge bases available over the Internet.

Current limitations soon will be overcome with new innovations. For example, mDevices will have beaming capabilities that will enable a clinician to project and type on the keyboard on a table or flat surface in the exam room, erasing the limitations of the device's small keyboard. Similarly, instead of viewing photos and videos on the device's small screen, these will be projected on walls or wireless monitors, creating professional theaters, where specialists will be able to gather in real time to view, discuss, and assess a patient, not just within a medical center setting but across settings or even across the world.

New functions will become more important. Consider picture taking and viewing. Physicians already can view x-rays, radiographs, and EKG strips on their mDevices, and patients with dermatologic conditions are sending pictures of their changing conditions to their providers, in many instances eliminating the necessity of office visits. Periodic and 24/7 monitoring of such signs as heart rhythm and blood pressure will become more mainstream, enabling earlier and more effective intervention. Much of this was unthinkable in the 1990s, but such applications will be increasingly adopted as their impact on healthcare is recognized and as patients become more educated about and involved in their health and disease management. Examples of new and evolving uses of mDevices include:

- Adapting a small ultrasound to interface with a mobile phone, allowing a patient to be scanned at home or elsewhere and sending the data wirelessly for evaluation by physicians with large screens

- Real-time, remote monitoring of intrapartum fetal heart tracing and uterine tonometry

- Using mobile phones as tactile listening aids for the deaf by converting voice received by the mobile phone's microphone into vibration applied to the skin

- Enhancing cell phones that have built-in cameras so that they can be used to do bacterial counts and other lab tests on bodily fluids, sending data to a remote computer, which analyzes the data and reports back by text message

Given these trends and innovations, and others we cannot yet anticipate, there is no question that the use of mDevices will continue to expand. There will be few people who do not have at least one mobile device, and more and more will give up their landlines. Further, those who do not buy the newest device every 12 to 18 months or so will fall behind in their professional capabilities and their social networking habits.

How mDevices Will Change Healthcare

This new era of mobile communication will change healthcare. Communications describing the observations of daily living (ODLs) will lead to new patterns of office visits. Patients are already researching signs, symptoms, conditions, and diseases on the Internet, and increasingly they will not accept a physician's advice without seeking this second opinion, which is available 24/7 at no additional cost. They also will be emboldened to question their physician when their research findings conflict with or supplement his recommendations. The cell phone will enable patients to access such information in concert with their physician, before leaving his office, perhaps even before leaving the exam room, thus further enabling point-of-care discussion with their physician about the advice their second opinion offers. Postvisit research will be followed up with real-time conversations with their physician through mDevice voice or data transmissions.

Physicians will have applets on their mDevice that will guide them through the care process. Indeed, some visionaries predict that the cell phone will move from being viewed as a "forbidden gadget to the most prized tool for every physician." Additionally, the next few years are expected to bring advanced, secure e-mail communication into healthcare, replacing older, more cumbersome, and less secure solutions (Waegemann 2009d).

Mobile phones will change healthcare far beyond such communication options. Future mDevices also will serve as the following:

- Identification devices that contain software for encryption and hold the key for accessing information

- General electronic keys used to open, turn on, and turn off doors and systems, such as security alarms, and specialized electronic keys that "break the glass" in emergency situations

- Remote controls for operating TVs, heating and air conditioning systems, stoves, and lights, including remote monitoring systems that, for example, can administer glucose when a diabetic patient's blood sugar falls below a certain level

- Electronic file cabinets that manage a mixture of direct data storage on the device and access to the wealth of other data via the Internet, as well as to a provider system's VPN, with access controlled via electronic keys that determine authorization by person, role, or circumstances

- Reminder systems that encourage a person to take his medication, to eat healthier, to live healthier, to comply more with specific cultural rules, and to behave in a more healthy fashion

- Monitors that report locations and activities and even may restrict the area within which the Alzheimer patient, for example, can walk. Many mDevices already have this fencing function built in but not yet activated.

Certainly, as demonstrated throughout this text, many leaders within the healthcare community see mHealth as an important stimulant toward patient-centric healthcare and as an enabler of participatory health. Dr. Jay Sanders of The Global Telemedicine Group argues that we should not be talking about mHealth but rather about bringing "the exam room to the patient" and "the collective experience of the practitioner to the patient's bedside." He also says, "We must migrate from a system based on episodic or periodic evaluation to one that provides continuous assessment" (Sanders 2009). The mDevice is the enabler that can move us toward these goals.

Yet the biggest change is still in its embryonic stage and will not have a real effect for the next year or two: Wireless connectivity in, or in proximity to, our bodies to capture vital signs, to transmit chemical processes from inside our bodies, and to report on our cellular functions. Such data will be captured from wearable items such as shirts, shoes, and clothing or from smart band aids, pills with wireless transmission, and implanted devices.

In some ways, the current trend of medicine is daunting. Within the next decade or so, medicine will revolutionize itself. Participatory health and the enabling mHealth technologies will be joined by miracles created by nanotechnology and personalized medicine. Disruptive, new, and exploding ways of enabling and accessing health information will make all these changes possible.

Challenges of the Future

At the same time, the increasing use of wireless devices may present some facilities with limits such as "brownouts" when no one can communicate internally or externally with the organization. Is this just a frightening thought or is it a real possibility? Certainly, there is enough concern that efforts to predict, avoid, and recover from such instances are being given more attention. Privacy and confidentiality concerns increasingly will require patients and providers—and HIM and other professionals—to work cooperatively to ensure that PHI is secure. Just as credit card companies and banks are working with their online customers to monitor their accounts more frequently and effectively than in the past in order to avoid fraudulent charges and transfer of funds, healthcare stakeholders must work together to avoid and quickly remedy unauthorized access to and use of personal health information.

Impact on HIM

When some medical informatics experts predicted in the 1980s that the implementation of EMRs would diminish the work of health information management, many believed this meant replacing transcriptionists with structured, direct data entry and diminishing the need for and responsibilities of HIM professionals. Those expectations generally have been wrong. The impact of digital communication and of the Internet on the role of HIM professionals cannot be compared with that on bank tellers who have largely been replaced by ATM machines or with that of airline check-in agents who are already being replaced by self check-in kiosks, which in turn, are being replaced by mDevice check-in, including boarding passes embedded in the mDevice, thus eliminating paper and the printing process as well.

While other modes of healthcare documentation have been adopted (or adapted) to some degree, there has been little effect on transcription quantity. In fact, more clinicians are acknowledging the need for and value of transcription, especially where free text cannot be replaced by structured data entry, thus expressing the recognition that transcription professionals have long sought. The appeal of mDevice applications that facilitate speech recognition (front end or back end) and structured data entry in concert with transcription, is expected to grow, thus creating the important responsibility for HIM professionals of managing these new hybrid forms of point-of-care and remote documentation and assuring their integration into EMRs and/or paper records.

The reality is that, just as EMRs have expanded and improved the role and status of HIM professionals, mDevices present the profession with great opportunities. Many new challenges will need to be mastered, as the role of HIM professionals expands to include communication management as well as information management. Their connections with both clinicians and patients are likely to expand as they assist each with research of, access to, and coordination of health and disease information as well as improved patient-provider communications. Likewise, their partnership with IT will grow, as it relies on specialists in that field to provide the technology necessary to achieve the full potential services that mDevices can provide, while assuring the confidentiality, privacy, and security of PHI. Such concerns also will create a stronger affiliation between HIMs and legal counsel as well as with C-level executives. Again, the greatest opportunities will be available to those HIM professionals who early on become actively involved in anticipating, designing, preparing for, and implementing these changes being stimulated by mDevices, mHealth, and participatory health.

A Sample Policies and Procedures Related to mHealth

As described in the main text, mHealth creates a range of new challenges to data integrity, security, authentication, and confidentiality of information. Thus, it is recommended that HIM professionals, in concert with legal counsel and others as designated by the enterprise, prepare policies that address the use of mHealth systems in their provider settings. The purpose of the following sample policies is not to guide HIM professionals toward restricting the use of mDevices but rather toward their legal, appropriate, and efficient use within the guidelines for data integrity and security associated with health information management

It must be kept in mind that these sample policies and procedures are just that— samples. It is essential that each institution's circumstances, needs, goals, and organizational strategy be taken into account as the devices are considered for adoption. Further, legal counsel must be consulted to ensure compliance with all applicable federal and state, as well as with other institutional, policies and procedures. Other appropriate personnel, including information technology and security personnel, should also participate in their development and adoption. It may be, too, that already existing policies and procedures related to protecting PHI, particularly those related to electronic medical records (for example, remote access to PHI), can be modified to incorporate mHealth considerations. Finally, additional policies and procedures may warrant development.

Definitions: For the purpose of the following sample policies, *mDevice* includes any mobile wireless device (for example, cell phone, smartphone, PDA, tablet, laptop, notebook, netbook, USB drive, CD, or RFID tag) that is or could be used to store, access, control, record, transmit, or otherwise utilize any PHI or other specified institutional information asset. *mHealth application* includes any health-related electronic application that is stored, accessed, transmitted, controlled, or otherwise utilized on or through such a mobile device.

Sample Policy – Adopting and Implementing mDevices and mHealth Applications

Purpose: The purpose of this policy is to provide guidance on the selection and implementation of mDevices and mHealth applications in healthcare environments.

Policy: In order to protect the integrity, legality and quality of care of storage, transmission, and retrieval of PHI, the adoption and implementation of mDevices and mHealth system applications must comply with all applicable state and federal regulations as well as institutional policies and procedures.

Procedure: HIM department works cooperatively with HIT department and department of bioengineering to:

1. Determine how to identify mHealth devices and mHealth applications that store, access, control, record, transmit, or otherwise utilize PHI and the degree to which they do so.

2. Determine how to protect the security and confidentiality of PHI on mDevices by implementing the necessary policies and procedures to assure security and confidentiality.

3. Determine who in what roles will be authorized to use these mDevices and mHealth applications and the degree to which such utilization will be restricted for certain categories of personnel and certain individuals and/or certain areas within or external to the facility.

4. Develop guidelines for such usage and disseminate these guidelines to authorized users as well as those who are restricted, in whole or in part, from such usage.

5. Document that these guidelines are received, reviewed, understood, and agreed to.

6. Conduct educational programs on the utilization of these devices and applications so as to protect the security and confidentiality of PHI.

7. Monitor the administration of these guidelines as well as the security and confidentiality abilities of the mDevices and mHealth applications.

8. Develop and disseminate a corrective action plan for instances in which the guidelines are infringed.

9. Establish and disseminate information on sanctions for infringements that lead to compromise and apply the sanctions appropriately.

10. Review and update related policies and procedures at least semiannually and on an ad hoc basis as required.

Sample Policy – Auditing mDevices and mHealth Applications

Purpose: The purpose of this policy is to provide guidance on the audits required for mHealth devices and applications.

Policy: In order to protect the integrity of the health information record and the PHI it contains and to provide quality patient care, mHealth systems accessing PHI should be used in compliance with all applicable state and federal regulations as well as institutional policies and procedures. Noncompliant use of mHealth functionalities is considered a sanctionable offense in accordance with the organizational policies.

Procedure: HIM Department works cooperatively with HIT department to:

1. Determine how to identify mHealth devices and mHealth applications that are to be audited.

2. Maintain an inventory of all such mHealth devices and mHealth applications, identifying types, versions, users, and purposes.

3. Test mHealth applications prior to implementation and prior to version updates.

4. Determine how and when audits will be conducted, including who will perform them, their frequency, the time period they cover, their sample size, and outcome indicators.

5. Design a corrective action plan based on findings.

Sample Policy: Authorization and Authentication of mDevice and mHealth Application Users

Purpose: The purpose of this policy is to provide guidance on user authorization and authentication in regards to mDevices and mHealth applications.

Policy: In order to protect PHI and the legality of information systems, as well as to protect institutional assets, mDevice and mHealth application access to PHI must require user authentication and must confirm access authorization before such access is granted. Access rights must be clearly defined and communicated to each potential user and nonuser, with limitations and restrictions designed to assure that access can be totally restricted, totally allowed, allowed only in certain circumstances, or restricted to certain parts of the record. Noncompliant access is considered a sanctionable offense in accordance with the organizational policies.

Procedure: HIM department, working cooperatively with HIT in regards to technical implementation:

1. Identifies personnel who are authorized to use mDevices and mHealth applications to access PHI and other institutional assets. This is done both by category (for example, clinical, administrative) and by individual within each category, as appropriate, and defines the extent of such authorization.

2. Assures that the technology requirements to determine and provide or restrict authorization and authentication are consistent with the policy requirements, including "breaking the glass" in emergency circumstances.

3. Develops guidelines to support authorization and authentication of users.

4. Designs and assures implementation of an institutionwide educational program regarding these guidelines.

5. Advises personnel as to their authorization rights and authentication requirements and documents their acknowledgment of the same.

6. Monitors the administration of these guidelines as well as the processes for authorization and authentication.

7. Develops and disseminates a corrective action plan for instances in which the guidelines are infringed.

8. Designs and implements an audit program to assure authorization and authentication are appropriately assigned and utilized.

9. Establishes and disseminates information on sanctions for infringements related to authorization and authentication that lead to compromised PHI and applies the sanctions appropriately.

10. Reviews and updates related policies and procedures at least semiannually and on an ad hoc basis as required.

Sample Policy: Implementing an Electromagnetic Compatibility (EMC) Program

Purpose: The purpose of this policy is to provide guidance on the implementation of an electromagnetic compatibility program.

Policy: In order to protect patients, medical devices, and others against the potential electromagnetic interference of medical devices by the utilization of mDevices in healthcare institutions, an electromagnetic compatibility program shall be instituted.

Procedure: HIM department works cooperatively with HIT and bioengineering departments to assure implementation of the recommendations of the FDA, Association of Image and Information Management (AIIM), IEEE, and others. Background information can be found in the Mobile Healthcare Alliance's (MoHCA) White Paper: Management of Wireless EMC in the Healthcare Environment (MoHCA 2004; available from the mHealth Initiative www.mhealthinitiative. org) and in ISO/TR Technical Report 21730:2006(E): Health Informatics—Use of mobile wireless communication and computing technology in healthcare facilities—Recommendations for electromagnetic compatibility (management of unintentional electromagnetic interference) with mobile devices (ISO 2006).

Sample Policy: Patient Authorization to Communicate By Electronic Means

Purpose: The purpose of this policy is to establish and implement institutional policies defining how a patient's authorization for eCommunications (for example, e-mail, text messaging, and instant messaging) will be determined, communicated to patients, and documented.

Policy: In order to protect patient rights, including the rights to confidentiality and privacy, patients shall be advised of their options for electronic communication, including the right to refuse or limit such options.

Procedure: The HIM department will work with the legal department to:

1. Determine whether the use of eCommunications with patients will be on an opt-in or an opt-out basis: Will the patient be required to document such authorization (opt in) before the enterprise can or will communicate with him electronically? Or, will the absence of objections or restrictions be considered authorization, so that only if the patient explicitly withholds such authorization (opts out)? Will eCommunication be restricted? Will the patient's initiation of electronic communications be considered a form of opt-in? Will the opt-in/opt-out policy vary by type of eCommunication (email, text messaging, instant messaging, and so on) and/or be dependent on its content (for example, allowing administrative eCommunications on an opt-out basis but requiring opt-in for PHI-related eCommunications)?

2. Develop documents that communicate to patients the institution's policies regarding their rights related to electronic communications, in accordance with the conclusions reached in step 1 above, including the risks to confidentiality or privacy that such media may entail.

3. Develop releases/authorizations that patients are to sign documenting their being informed of their rights and, where authorization is required, their decisions regarding the use of eCommunications, including any limitations that they want applied to such communications (for example, the exclusion or inclusion of all or certain types of PHI communications).

4. Develop educational programs to communicate to appropriate personnel (for example, admitting, registration, clinicians) the policies in place and how to administer them.

5. Maintain documentation of each patient's opt-in/opt-out status.

6. Monitor the administration of these policies.

Sample Policy: Audit Trails of Access to PHI through mDevices and mHealth Applications

Purpose: The purpose of this policy is to assure that audit trails are instituted to document authorized and unauthorized access to PHI through mDevices and mHealth applications as well as attempts that are blocked or denied.

Policy: In order to document access to PHI through mDevices and mHealth applications, a process must be in place to create an audit trail of all such successful or denied access to PHI. This audit trail shall identify the entity (person or system) achieving or being blocked from such access and what information was accessed or denied, and it shall include a date/time stamp identifying when the access was made or denied.

Procedure: The HIM department shall work with the IT department and security officer to:

1. Design audit trails for access to PHI through mDevices, including data to be included in each audit point.

2. Educate personnel regarding the need for and utilization of audit trails for access to PHI through mDevices.

3. Establish a calendar for generating routine audit reports and review the same in a timely manner.

4. Monitor the audit trails on a random basis as well.

5. Be automatically notified of denied access as well as unauthorized breaches.

6. Develop and disseminate a corrective action plan for instances in which the audit trail identifies denials or breaches.

7. Determine action to be taken as a result of denials or breaches.

8. Review and update audit trail policies and procedures at least semiannually and on an ad hoc basis as required.

Sample Policy: Clearing the Memory of mDevices

Purpose: The purpose of this policy is to protect patient confidentiality and privacy against access through mDevices that are stolen or lost as well as those that are no longer in use or are being transferred to another user.

Policy: In order to protect against unauthorized access to PHI in the event an mDevice is lost, stolen, no longer in use, or transferred to another user, a process shall be in place requiring notification regarding such instances and assuring that the memory of such mDevices is cleared.

Procedure: The HIM department, in cooperation with the IT department shall:

1. Assure that instructions for clearing the memory of each type of mDevice under the institution's jurisdiction are maintained in print or electronic form or both. Such instructions should include both in-hand and remote clearance of the memory.

2. In instances where such mDevices do not have the capacity for remotely clearing the memory, the addition of an application on the device shall be required before storage of PHI on the device is authorized, and instructions related to such applications shall be cataloged and maintained.

3. Develop a policy that requires mDevice users to notify the HIM and HIT departments immediately when an mDevice that contains or allows access to PHI is lost or stolen or when the user is replacing the device or passing it on to someone else. Such notification should identify the degree to which PHI is on the device and/or its applications and whether the user has cleared the memory, including PHI. Failed attempts for clearing must also be reported.

4. Designate personnel in the HIM and/or HIT department responsible for confirming memory clearance by the user and for clearing the memory when the user either has not done so or his attempts have failed.

5. Assure that stolen mDevices are reported to law enforcement.

6. Maintain documentation of all memory clearance activities, specifying device and/applications, user, types of PHI cleared, dates, and times any special circumstances and any failed attempts.

7. In the event that security of PHI has been breached, notification of patients and authorities shall be done in accordance with institutional guidelines and federal (including HIPAA and ARRA) and state guidelines.

Sample Policy: Picture-taking with mDevices

Purpose: The purpose of this policy is to protect patient confidentiality and privacy against unauthorized picture-taking with mDevices.

Policy: In order to protect patient confidentiality, all employees, contractors, and volunteers must be advised that taking pictures of patients must be restricted to pictures for clinical use and that sanctions will be applied in the event unauthorized pictures of patients are taken.

Procedure: The HIM department will work cooperatively with the legal department to:

1. Develop policies regarding authorized and unauthorized picture-taking of patients. These policies should:

   - Define authorized picture-taking for clinical purposes, including who is authorized to take such pictures.

   - Restrict all other picture-taking and all other personnel from taking pictures of patients.

   - Restrict the use of authorized pictures from other uses.

   - Identify sanctions for infringements of the policy.

2. Develop an educational plan for advising all personnel about authorized and restricted picture-taking of patients.

3. Monitor the administration of these policies.

4. Develop and disseminate a corrective action plan for instances in which the policy is infringed.

5. Identify sanctions for infringements and apply the sanctions appropriately.

6. Review and update related policies and procedures at least semiannually and on an ad hoc basis as required, including requiring acknowledgment of updated policies through new signed agreements.

Sample Security Agreement – Regarding mDevice Use

Each employee, contractor, volunteer, student, or other person affiliated with any healthcare institution is required by law and institutional policies to commit to protecting and not violating the confidentiality and security of PHI, as evidenced by signature of a security agreement. Such agreements should be amended to specifically address mDevices and mHealth applications, whether used within or outside the institution's premises, and they should reference definitions of mDevices and mHealth applications as indicated in the sample agreement.

Note: This sample form should not be used without review by your organization's legal counsel to ensure compliance with federal, local, and state laws and institutional policies and procedures.

Employee/Contractor/Student/Volunteer Nondisclosure Agreement

[*Name of healthcare provider*] has a legal and ethical responsibility to safeguard the privacy of all patients and protect the confidentiality of their health information. In the course of my employment/contractor work/assignment at [*name of healthcare provider*], I may come into possession of confidential patient information, even though I may not be directly involved in providing patient services.

I understand that such information must be maintained in the strictest confidence. As a condition of my employment/contract /assignment, I hereby agree that, unless directed by my authorized supervisor, I will not at any time during or after my employment/contract work/ assignment with [*name of healthcare provider*] disclose any patient information to any person whatsoever or permit any person whatsoever to examine or make copies of any patient reports or other documents prepared by me, coming into my possession, or under my control or use patient information, other than as necessary in the course of my employment/assignment. When patient information must be discussed with other healthcare practitioners in the course of my work/assignment, I will use discretion to ensure that such conversations cannot be overheard by others who are not involved in the patient's care.

Further, I understand that I may access, record, and/or store patient information on a mobile device (mDevice) and/or mobile health (mHealth) application (mDevice and mHealth application as defined below) only to the extent to which I am authorized to do so and only in a manner consistent with federal and state regulations and institutional policies and procedures relevant to the protection of the confidentiality, privacy, and security of protected health information (PHI). I understand that violation of this agreement may result in corrective action, up to and including discharge.

> **mDevice:** Any mobile wireless device (for example, cell phone, smartphone, PDA, tablet, laptop, notebook, netbook, USB drive, CD, RFID tag, or other mobile computing or communication device) that is or could be used to store, access, control, record, transmit, or otherwise utilize any PHI or other specified institutional information asset.

> **mHealth Application:** Any health-related electronic application that is stored, accessed, transmitted , controlled, or otherwise utilized on or through a mobile device.

Signature of Employee/Contractor/Student/Volunteer

Date

Source: Adapted from AHIMA 2003

APPENDIX **B** Resources

AHIMA. 2009 (May). Sanction guidelines for privacy and security breaches. *Journal of AHIMA*. 80(5): 57–62.

AHIMA e-HIM Work Group on Medical Identity Theft. 2008. Mitigating medical identity theft. *Journal of AHIMA*. 79(7):63–69.

Dinh, A. K. 2009 (January). Securing portable devices. *Journal of AHIMA*. 80(1): 56–57.

Parmiagiani, J. 2009 (April). Webinar: Managing the challenges of portable devices.

Southerton, L. 2009 (June). Mobile device use, reuse, and disposal. *Journal of AHIMA*. 78(6): 68–70.

REFERENCES

3G Americas. 2008 (December). World wireless market: World cellular subscriptions.
http://www.3gamericas.org/index.cfm?fuseaction=page&pageid=565

Adler, P. 2009 (April 15). Breach notification involving protected health information.

AHIMA e-HIM Personal Health Record Work Group. 2005. The role of the personal health record in the EHR. *Journal of AHIMA* 76(7):64A-D.

AHIMA e-HIM Work Group on Medical Identity Theft. 2008. Mitigating medical identity theft. *Journal of AHIMA* 79(7):63–69.

AirMagnet. 2009. White paper: Impact of healthcare applications on WLAN mobility. Sunnyvale, CA: AirMagnet.

Albin, S. 2009. Physician ethics on Facebook. Facebook.
http://www.facebook.com/group.php?gid=37882434106

American Health Information Management Association. 2003. Practice Brief: Employee/student/volunteer nondisclosure agreement. *Journal of AHIMA* 74(6), 64B.

American Health Information Management Association. 2008. The power of PHR. *AHIMA Advantage* 12(3).

ASTM. 2007. E2553-07 Standard guide for implementation of a voluntary universal healthcare identification (VUHID) system. West Conshohocken, PA: ASTM International.
http://www.astm.org/Standards/E2553.htm

ASTM. 2007. E1714-07 Standard guide for properties of a universal healthcare identifier (UHID). West Conshohocken, PA: ASTM International.
http://www.astm.org/Standards/E1714.htm

ASTM. 2005. E236-05 Standard specification for continuity of care record (CCR). West Conshohocken, PA: ASTM International.
http://astm.org/Standards/E2369.htm

Beaulieu, L. 2009 (March 31). Clinical grade requirements to enable a mobile health and advanced workflow environment. mHealth Initiative Seminar. Boston: mHealth Initiative.
http://www.slideshare.net/mHealthInitiative/clinical-grade-reqmtsto-enable-mobile-healthm-h-i-i2009-final

Blumberg, S.J., J.V. Luke, G. Davidson, M.E. Davern, T.C. Yu, and K. Soderberg. 2009 (March 11). Wireless substitution: State-level estimates from the National Health Interview, January–December 2007. National Health Statistics Reports, 14.

Brennan, P. 2009 (June 4). Project Health Design and mHealth. mHealth Initiative Seminar. Washington, DC: mHealth Initiative.

CDC Online Newsroom. 2009 (March 11). Wireless-only phone use varies widely across United States. Atlanta: Centers for Disease Control and Prevention.
http://www.cdc.gov/media/pressrel/2009/r090311.htm

Chen, P. 2009 (June 11). Doctor and Patient: Medicine in the age of Twitter. *New York Times*.

Consensus Workgroup on Health Information Capture and Report Generation. 2002 (June). Healthcare documentation: A report on information capture and report generation. Newton, MA: Medical Records Institute.

Crick, T. 2009 (July 28). The Need for a M2M Secure Connectivity Platform. Fifth Annual Smart Services Leadership Summit, San Diego.

CTIA Media. 2008. Wireless quick facts. CTIA-The Wireless Association. http://www.ctia.org/media/industry_info/index.cfm/AID/10323

Davis, H. 2004. *Absolute Beginner's Guide to Wi-Fi Wireless Networking*. Toronto, Ontario: Que Publishing.

DesRoches, C.M., E.G. Campbell, S.R. Rao, K. Donelan, T.G. Ferris, A. Jha, R. Kaushal, D.E. Levy, S. Rosenbau, A.E. Shields, and D. Blumenthal. 2008 (July 3). Electronic health records in ambulatory care—a national survey of physicians. *New England Journal of Medicine*. http://content.nejm.org/cgi/content/full/359/1/50

Dinh, A.K. 2009. Securing Portable Devices. *Journal of AHIMA* 80(1), 56–57.

EMI/EMC Standards Organizations. (1997–2008). RADIOING.com. http://www.radioing.com/eengineer/emc-orgs.html

Fox, S. 2009 (June). The social life of health information: Americans' pursuit of health takes place within a widening network of both online and offline resources. Pew Internet & American Life Project. http://www.pewinternet.org/Reports/2009/8-The-Social-Life-of-Health-Information. aspx?r=1

Global Patient Identifiers, Inc. 2009. http://www.gpii.info/

Gow, J. 2009 (August 11). Securing Mobile Devices in the Enterprise. ISSA Web Conference— the Truth about Securing Mobile Devices.

Graves, A.F., B. Wallace, S. Periyalwar, and C. Riccardi. 2005 (October). Clinical grade— a foundation for healthcare communications networks. Fifth International Workshop on Design of Reliable Communication Networks. Institute of Electrical and Electronics Engineers (IEEE).

Health on the Internet Foundation. 2008. The HON Code in brief. http://www.hon.ch/HONcode/Patients/Conduct.html

Hendrich, A., M. Chow, B.A. Skiercynzki, L. Zhengqiang. 2008. A 36-hospital time and motion study: How do nurses spend their time? *The Permanente Journal* 12(3):25–34.

ISO. 2006. ISO/TR Technical Report 21730:2006(E): *Health Informatics—Use of mobile wireless communication and computing technology in healthcare facilities—Recommendations for electromagnetic compatibility (management of unintentional electromagnetic interference) with mobile devices*. International Organization for Standardization (ISO).

Kane, B. and D. Sands. 1998. Guidelines for clinical use of electronic mail with patients. *Journal of the American Medical Informatics Association* 5(1):104–111.

Kolakowski, N. 2009 (April 13). Google Health accused of inaccuracy in electronic medical records. Healthcare IT—eWeek. http://www.eweek.com/c/a/Health-Care-IT/Google-Health-Accused-of-Inaccuracy-in-Electronic-Medical-Records-603668/

Lindstrom, P. 2009 (August 11). Protecting good things in small packages. ISSA Web Conference—the Truth about Securing Mobile Devices.

May, C. 2009 (September 3). Email message to editor.

McLeod, R.P. 2009 (March 31). Using Mobile Technology to Transform Nursing Practice. mHealth Initiative Seminar. Boston: mHealth Initiative.
http://www.slideshare.net/mHealthInitiative/nursestechnologymhiseminarmcleod

Miller, C.C. and M. Richtel. 2009 (June 22). Investors bet on payments via cellphone. *New York Times.*
http://www.nytimes.com/2009/06/22/technology/22pay.html?hpw

Miller-Jacobs, H. 2009. (March 31). Usability: A critical component of the mHealth Initiative. mHealth Initiative Seminar. Boston: mHealth Initiative.

Mobile Healthcare Alliance (MoHCA). 2004. White paper: Management of wireless EMC in the healthcare environment. Boston: Mobile Healthcare Alliance (MoHCA).

National Alliance for Health Information Technology, 2008 (April 28). Report to the Office of the National Coordinator for Health Information Technology on defining key health information technology terms. Chicago: NAHIT.
http://www.nahit.org/images/pdfs/HITTermsFinalReport_051508.pdf

Parmigiani, J.C. 2009 (April 24). AHIMA Webinar: The challenge of managing portable devices.

PinStack.com. 2005. List of acronyms and text messaging shorthand.
http://forums.pinstack.com/showthread.php?t=609 or http://www.netlingo.com/ acronyms.php

Pringle, J. 2008 (May 10). Saving lives in San Diego. TEPR 2008 Conference. Fort Lauderdale: Medical Records Institute.

Quinn, C.C., S.S. Clough, J.M. Minor, D. Lender, M.C. Okafor, and A.Gruber-Baldini. 2008. WellDoc™ mobile diabetes management randomized control trial: Change in clinical and behavioral outcomes and patient and physician satisfaction. *Diabetes Technology & Therapeutics* 10(3).

Rothstein, J. and L. Ricciardi. 2009 (July 27). A pocket full of ODLs. Project HealthDesign.
http://www.typepad.com/services/trackback/6a00df35210d198834011572310529970b

Sabett, R.V. 2009 (August 11). Legal Concerns in the Mobile World. ISSA Web Conference—the Truth about Securing Mobile Devices.

Sanders, J. 2009 (June 4). So…where do we go from here? mHealth Initiative Seminar. Washington, DC: mHealth Initiative.

SearchMobileComputing.com. Personal area network. 2008 (October 17).
http://searchmobilecomputing.techtarget.com/sDefinition/0,,sid40_gci546288,00.html#

Stern, E. 2009 (June 4). The patient's back-up brain: A mobile health future. mHealth Initiative Seminar. Washington, DC: mHealth Initiative.

Stross, R. 2008 (December 26). What carriers aren't eager to tell you about texting. *New York Times.*
http://www.nytimes.com/2008/12/28/business/28digi.html?_r=1

Tewson, K., and S. Riley. 2008. Security watch: A guide to wireless security. Microsoft TechNet.
http://207.46.16.252/en-us/magazine/2005.11.securitywatch.aspx

Waegemann, C.P. 2008. Presentation: Overlapping eHealth and mHealth. Boston: Medical Records Institute.

Waegemann, C.P. 2009a (March 31). The mHealth Revolution. mHealth Initiative Seminar. Boston: mHealth Initiative.
http://www.slideshare.net/mHealthInitiative/m-health-c-p-w

Waegemann, C.P. 2009b (March 31). Proposed mHealth Project. mHealth Initiative Seminar. Boston: mHealth Initiative.
http://www.slideshare.net/mHealthInitiative/proposed-m-health-project-c-p-w

Waegemann, C.P. 2009c (March–May). Personal communication with author.

Waegemann, C.P. 2009d (June). Personal communication with author.

Waegemann, C.P. and C. Tessier (2009a). Traditional and new communications between patients and healthcare providers. Boston: mHealth Initiative.

Waegemann, C.P. and C. Tessier (2009b). Traditional and new research options for clinicians. Boston: mHealth Initiative.

Waegemann, C.P. and C. Tessier (2009c). How healthcare documentation is changing. Boston: mHealth Initiative.

Wallace, B. and C. Graves. 2006. Healthcare technology standards—Driven by solutions to clinicians' needs. Nortel.
http://grouper.ieee.org/groups/hit/files/Wallace-IEEE_Clinical_grade_presentation_v4.pdf

Wenner, M. 2008 (November 21). Fact or fiction: Cell phones can cause brain cancer. *Scientific American*.
http://www.scientificamerican.com/article.cfm?id=fact-or-fiction-cell-phones-can-cause-brain-cance.

Wernick, A.S. 2007. Connectivity, privacy, and liability: What medical professionals must consider. *Journal of AHIMA*. 78(4):64–65.

INDEX